Atlas of Radiographic Anatomy of the Horse

Atlas der Röntgenanatomie des Pferdes

ATLAS
DER RÖNTGENANATOMIE
DES PFERDES

Dr. H. SCHEBITZ

o. ö. Professor, Vorstand der Chirurgischen
Universitäts-Tierklinik
München

Dr. H. WILKENS

o. Professor, Direktor des Anatomischen
Instituts der Tierärztlichen Hochschule
Hannover

Dritte, neubearbeitete Auflage

Mit 45 Röntgenbildern, 45 Röntgenskizzen und 38 Lagerungsskizzen

1978

VERLAG PAUL PAREY · BERLIN UND HAMBURG

W. B. SAUNDERS COMPANY · PHILADELPHIA UND TORONTO

ATLAS OF RADIOGRAPHIC ANATOMY OF THE HORSE

Dr. H. SCHEBITZ

o. ö. Professor, Vorstand der Chirurgischen
Universitäts-Tierklinik
München

Dr. H. WILKENS

o. Professor, Direktor des Anatomischen
Instituts der Tierärztlichen Hochschule
Hannover

Third revised edition

With 45 Radiographs, 45 Radiographic Sketches, and 38 Positioning-Drawings

1978

VERLAG PAUL PAREY · BERLIN AND HAMBURG

W. B. SAUNDERS COMPANY · PHILADELPHIA AND TORONTO

Bilingual published in German and English by Verlag Paul Parey, Berlin and Hamburg, Germany.
Adresses: Lindenstrasse 44—47, 1000 Berlin 61; Spitalerstrasse 12, 2000 Hamburg 1.
Sales Rights for United States of America, Canada, Latin America, Australia and New Zealand: W. B. Saunders Company, Philadelphia and Toronto.

The 1st edition was published 1967 under the title
"Atlas of Radiographic Anatomy of Dog and Horse"
ISBN 3-489-74816-6;

the 2nd edition was published 1973 under the title
"Atlas of Radiographic Anatomy of Dog and Horse"
ISBN 3-489-75116-7.

Beginning with the 3rd edition, there is a new arrangement: This volume deals with the "Radiographic Anatomy of the Horse" and the volume published in 1977 with the "Radiographic Anatomy of the Dog and Cat".

Zweisprachig herausgegeben in deutscher und englischer Sprache vom Verlag Paul Parey, Berlin und Hamburg, Germany.
Anschriften: Lindenstraße 44—47, 1000 Berlin 61; Spitalerstraße 12, 2000 Hamburg 1.
Vertriebsrechte für USA, Kanada, Süd-Amerika, Australien und Neuseeland: W. B. Saunders Company, Philadelphia und Toronto.

Die 1. Auflage erschien 1967 unter dem Titel
„Atlas der Röntgenanatomie von Hund und Pferd"
ISBN 3-489-74816-6.

Die 2. Auflage erschien 1973 unter dem Titel
„Atlas der Röntgenanatomie von Hund und Pferd"
ISBN 3-489-75116-7.

Von der 3. Auflage an gilt eine andere Einteilung: Dieser Band umfaßt die „Röntgenanatomie des Pferdes", der 1977 erschienene Band die „Röntgenanatomie von Hund und Katze".

Atlas of Radiographic Anatomy of the Horse   ISBN 0-7216-7964-1
Cover and jacket design: CHRISTIAN HONIG, Neuwied (Rhein)

© 1978 by Paul Parey, Berlin and Hamburg, Germany
Addresses: Lindenstraße 44—47, 1000 Berlin 61; Spitalerstraße 12, 2000 Hamburg 1
Printed in Germany by Felgentreff & Goebel KG, 1000 Berlin 61, Germany

ISBN 3-489-69316-7 Verlag Paul Parey, Berlin and Hamburg
ISBN 0-7216-7964-1 W. B. Saunders Company, Philadelphia and Toronto

Preface to the third edition

In the present third edition the radiographic anatomy of the cat has been included. In this way the subject matter could be arranged more meaningfully for use in practice in an "Atlas of the Radiographic Anatomy of the Horse" and an "Atlas of the Radiographic Anatomy of the Dog and Cat". Nevertheless, certain chapters still need to be supplemented.

During the past few years the nomenclature of Nomina Anatomica Veterinaria (NAV) has been adopted universally and included in textbooks. It was therefore decided to discontinue the listing of terms commonly used in German and English.

Thanks are due to Professor Dr. J. M. W. LE ROUX, Onderstepoort, South Africa, and Dr. Dr. V. SOKOLOVSKY, Chicago, U.S.A., for their kind advice and assistance in preparing the english texts.

We are deeply indebted to the following members of our staff: Mrs. B. GROSS and Mrs. U. LANDHERR for the carefully prepared radiographs; Mrs. R. ROCHNER, graphic artist, for the meticulously prepared radiographic sketches and the positioning-drawings; Mrs. M. L. MEINECKE, Dr. W. MÜNSTER, academic director, Dr. (Mrs.) U. MATIS, Dr. (Mrs.) I. GUNSSER and Mrs. G. HOLZBAUER for their dedicated and kind cooperation in all the preliminary preparations prior to publication.

We should like to express our sincere gratitude towards DDr. h. c. F. GEORGI, co-owner of the Paul Parey Publishing Company and his production manager, Mr. E. TOPSCHOWSKY for the excellent and careful production of the book. They have submitted to our demands at all times with great understanding.

It is to be hoped that the Atlas of the Radiographic Anatomy of the Horse will be well received.

Munich and Hanover, in the winter of 1977/78　　　　　　　　　　　　HORST SCHEBITZ, HELMUT WILKENS

Preface to the first edition

To be proficient in the field of radiologic diagnosis, one must be familiar with the radiographic anatomy. Until recently, there has been no book providing the student or the insufficiently experienced veterinarian with the basic anatomy necessary for the interpretation of radiographs. As an introduction into this special field is not possible without abundant illustrations, clinician and anatomist have cooperated to compile an Atlas of the Radiographic Anatomy of the Dog and Horse. This atlas was written for the practising veterinarian; consequently, it also contains instructions for radiographic technique which, with experience and the proper equipment, should produce consistently good radiographs.

In order to find access to a greater number of readers, the atlas is published in German and English.

Our special thanks go to Dr. Dr. V. SOKOLOVSKY, Chicago, U. S. A., for the translation of the legends to the positioning-drawings and consultation on all other aspects of the translation, and to Mr. G. W. O. SPECKMANN and Mr. G. L. YOUNG for their active participation in the translation of the legends to the drawings of the radiographs. We are indebted to Mr. W. HEINEMANN for consultation with respect to the illustrations, to Mr. G. KAPITZKE for the positioning-drawings and radiographic sketches, to Miss D. ABRAMOWSKI and Mrs. G. BUERKLE for the labelling of the drawings of the radiographs, to Mr. G. OBERST for the copies of the radiographs which were made with the greatest of care, and last but not least to Drs. W. ZEDLER, M. SASCHEK, H. WISSDORF, K. NEURAND, Chr. PAULICK, and also to the medical technicians Miss M. L. MEINECKE, Miss B. GROSS, and Miss A. VAN DER GROEBEN for their assistance in all preparatory work prior to printing.

Although the number of radiographs in this atlas has already been increased from 60 to 94, there are still individual chapters which call for improvement.

Our sincere thanks are due to the publishers, Paul Parey, for their understanding shown towards the inevitable increase in volume of the atlas, and for providing the fine reproductions of the radiographs. We hope that this atlas will be a useful addition to the veterinary medical literature.

Munich and Hanover, Summer of 1967　　　　　　　　　　　　HORST SCHEBITZ, HELMUT WILKENS

Vorwort zur dritten Auflage

In die vorliegende 3. Auflage konnte die Röntgenanatomie der Katze aufgenommen werden. Dadurch wurde eine für die tägliche Praxis zweckmäßige Aufteilung des Stoffes in einen „Atlas der Röntgenanatomie des Pferdes" und einen „Atlas der Röntgenanatomie von Hund und Katze" möglich. Keiner Erörterung bedarf es, daß trotzdem Wünsche nach Ergänzung einzelner Kapitel bleiben.

Im Laufe der letzten Jahre wurden die Termini technici der Nomina Anatomica Veterinaria weltweit in die Lehrbücher übernommen. Deshalb werden die bisher im Deutschen und Englischen üblichen Bezeichnungen nicht mehr aufgeführt.

Für die freundliche Beratung und die liebenswürdige Hilfe bei der Abfassung der englischen Texte danken wir Herrn Prof. Dr. J. M. W. Le Roux, Onderstepoort/Südafrika, und Herrn Dr. Dr. V. Sokolovsky, Chicago/USA.

Zu großem Dank sind wir unseren Mitarbeitern verpflichtet: Frau B. Gross und Frau U. Landherr für die mit großer Sorgfalt angefertigten Vorlagen; der Graphikerin Frau R. Rochner für die ausgezeichneten Röntgen- und die anschaulichen Lagerungsskizzen; Frau M. L. Meinecke, dem Akad. Direktor Herrn Dr. W. Münster, Frau Dr. U. Matis, Frau Dr. I. Gunsser und Frau G. Holzbauer für die gewissenhafte und freundliche Unterstützung bei allen vorbereitenden Arbeiten zur Drucklegung.

Dem Mitinhaber des Verlages Paul Parey, Herrn DDr. h. c. F. Georgi, und seinem Mitarbeiter, Herrn E. Topschowsky, danken wir für die hervorragende verlegerische Gestaltung und für das unseren Wünschen stets entgegengebrachte Verständnis.

Wir hoffen, daß der „Atlas der Röntgenanatomie des Pferdes" eine gute Aufnahme findet.

München und Hannover, im Winter 1977/78   Horst Schebitz, Helmut Wilkens

Vorwort zur ersten Auflage

Wenn man Röntgendiagnostik betreibt, ist es zweckmäßig, sich mit der Röntgenanatomie zu befassen. Auf diesem Spezialgebiet fehlten bislang Bücher, die dem Studierenden oder auch dem noch wenig mit der Röntgenologie vertrauten Tierarzt die normal-anatomischen Grundlagen für die Interpretation von Röntgenaufnahmen vermitteln. Da eine Einführung in dieses Fachgebiet nicht ohne vielseitiges Abbildungsmaterial erfolgen kann, haben Kliniker und Anatom gemeinsam einen Atlas der Röntgenanatomie von Hund und Pferd erstellt. Die Konzeption des vorliegenden Atlas ist auf die Belange der kurativen Praxis abgestimmt. Der Atlas enthält Hinweise für die Aufnahmetechnik, die bei gewisser Erfahrung und bei Verfügung über die notwendigen Geräte zu jederzeit reproduzierbaren Ergebnissen führen sollen.

Um einen möglichst großen Interessentenkreis zu gewinnen, erscheint der Atlas zweisprachig — deutsch und englisch.

Herrn Dr. Dr. V. Sokolovsky, Chicago/USA, sei an dieser Stelle unser besonderer Dank für die Übersetzung der Legenden zu den Lagerungsskizzen und für die Beratung in allen weiteren Fragen bei der Übersetzungsarbeit ausgesprochen. Ebenso gilt unser Dank den Herren G. W. O. Speckmann und G. L. Young für ihre tatkräftige Mithilfe bei der Übersetzung der Legenden zu den Röntgenskizzen, Herrn W. Heinemann für die Beratung bei der graphischen Gestaltung der Abbildungen, Herrn G. Kapitzke für die Ausführung der Lagerungszeichnungen und Röntgenskizzen, Fräulein D. Abramowski sowie Frau G. Bürkle für die Beschriftung der Röntgenskizzen, Herrn G. Oberst für die Vorlagen der Röntgenbilder, die er mit größter Sorgfalt angefertigt hat, und nicht zuletzt den Herren Drs. W. Zedler, M. Saschek, H. Wissdorf, K. Neurand und Frau Dr. Chr. Paulick sowie den med.-techn. Assistentinnen Fräulein M. L. Meinecke, Fräulein B. Gross und Fräulein A. van der Groeben für ihre freundliche Unterstützung bei allen vorbereitenden Arbeiten zur Drucklegung.

Obwohl gegenüber der ersten Planung die Zahl der Röntgenaufnahmen von 60 auf 94 erhöht wurde, bleiben noch immer Wünsche nach Ergänzung einzelner Kapitel.

Dem Verlag Paul Parey gebührt für das Verständnis der erforderlich gewordenen Umfangsvermehrung des Atlas, insbesondere aber auch für die Ausstattung mit der gelungenen Wiedergabe der Röntgenaufnahmen, unser aufrichtiger Dank.

Möge der Atlas allen Interessenten ein brauchbarer Ratgeber sein.

München und Hannover, im Sommer 1967   Horst Schebitz, Helmut Wilkens

Contents — Inhaltsverzeichnis

Einleitung

Die Gliederung des Atlas erfolgt bei den Aufnahmen von Skelett und Gelenken nach Körperregionen.

Die Röntgenaufnahmen wurden ausnahmslos an lebenden Pferden unter den für die Diagnostik zweckmäßigen Bedingungen angefertigt. Sie sind im Atlas als Negativ reproduziert. Die Abbildung im Buch entspricht mithin der im durchfallenden Licht zu betrachtenden Röntgenaufnahme. Bei der Reproduktion von Röntgenaufnahmen müssen wegen der großen Schwärzungsdifferenzen geringe Verluste an Details in Kauf genommen werden. Da die Röntgenskizzen nach dem Original bei durchfallendem Licht gezeichnet wurden, sind in einigen Skizzen Details enthalten, die in den Röntgenabbildungen beim Druck verlorengegangen sind.

Jede Röntgenaufnahme wird durch eine Bildunterschrift erklärt: Zunächst wird der Körperteil genannt; darauf folgen die Lage des Tieres bzw. Körperteils und schließlich die Richtung des Strahlengangs.

Weiterhin werden technische Daten angegeben: Blende, Filmmaterial, Folien und Einstellung. Dabei gelten folgende Abkürzungen: FFA = Fokus-Film-Abstand, kV = Kilovolt, mAs = Milliampère-Sekunden-Produkt.

Jede Röntgenabbildung wird durch eine Röntgenskizze erläutert, die Abbildungshinweise enthält. Dabei erfolgt keine Beschränkung auf bestimmte Details. Dadurch erscheinen manche der Skizzen auf den ersten Blick mit Abbildungshinweisen überladen. Der Vorteil der Skizzen ist aber darin zu sehen, daß die Röntgenaufnahmen frei von erklärenden Hinweisen bleiben.

Folgende Hinweise sind bei den Röntgenskizzen zu beachten:

* Soweit differenzierbar, und wenn in der Legende nicht besonders erwähnt, kennzeichnen Buchstaben und Zahlen mit hochgesetztem Strich (A′; 1′) filmferne Skeletteile.

** Bei Überlagerungen im Bereich der Gelenke sind die filmnahen Konturen durchgezogen, die filmfernen unterbrochen dargestellt.

Lagerungsskizzen veranschaulichen die Aufnahmetechnik mit der Fixierung des zu untersuchenden Tieres durch Hilfspersonen. Der Zentralstrahl ist durch eine gestrichelte Linie, seine Auftreffstelle am Tierkörper durch einen Punkt gekennzeichnet. Keiner Erörterung bedarf es, daß bei den Röntgenaufnahmen die Vorschriften über den Strahlenschutz zu berücksichtigen sind.

Im deutschen wie im englischen Sprachgebrauch werden ausschließlich Termini technici der Nomina Anatomica Veterinaria (1973) verwendet.

Richtungsbezeichnungen für den Strahlengang sind auf die Nomina Anatomica Veterinaria abgestimmt. Dabei sei auf die Publikation von Habel et al. (1963) verwiesen.

Als Abkürzungen gelten: A. = Arteria, V. = Vena, M. = Musculus, N. = Nervus.

Die Bibliographie berücksichtigt nur die Bücher der Veterinär-Anatomie bzw. Röntgenologie sowie Publikationen, die zur Erstellung des Atlas herangezogen wurden oder bei vorbereitenden Untersuchungen Berücksichtigung fanden.

Auf ein Sachregister wurde bewußt verzichtet, da dieses nur eine Wiederholung der Termini darstellen würde und andererseits zur Benutzung des Atlas für bestimmte röntgenologische Fragestellungen anatomische Grundkenntnisse vorausgesetzt werden dürfen.

Introduction

The radiographs of the skeleton and joints are arranged according to the body regions.

All radiographs were taken of live horses under conditions best suitable for diagnostic purposes. They are reproduced as negatives. The illustrations, therefore, correspond to radiographs viewed under trans-illumination. Because of considerable differences in blacking, some detail is lost in the process of reproduction. Since the sketches were drawn from the original radiographs, trans-illuminated, some of them show details which were lost during reproduction of the radiographs.

Each radiograph is provided with a legend: skeletal parts are mentioned first; this is followed by the position-in of the animal and the region for the body respectively and finally by the direction of the beam. Furthermore, technical data are provided: diaphragm, film, screen and setting.

The following abbreviations are used: FFD = Focus Film Distance, kV = Kilovoltage, mAs = Milliampère second.

A detailed sketch with references accompanies each radiograph. At first sight many of the sketches appear to be overcrowded with references, however, it has the advantage that radiographs remain free of inscriptions.

The following directions should be observed in connection with the X-ray sketches:

* As far as skeletal parts can be identified and if not specifically mentioned in the legends, prime letters and numerals with stroke (A′; 1′) refer to parts next to the tube.

** In the case of superimposition of contours in the joint regions, those next to the film are indicated by continuous lines, those next to tube by interrupted lines.

The drawings of the positioning illustrate the radiographic technique and the immobilisation of the animal. The central X-ray beam is shown by an interrupted line and the point of its impact on the body by a dot. Protective measures against radiation need hardly be mentioned.

The nomenclature used in this atlas is based on Nomina Anatomica Veterinaria (1973).

Directional terms for the X-ray beam are based on Nomina Anatomica Veterinaria. In this respect the reader is referred to the publication of HABEL et al. (1963).

Abbreviations: A. = Artery, V. = Vein, M. = Muscle, N. = Nerve.

In legends the official terms are not translated. Explanatory notes in German are translated.

The bibliography includes only those books and publications on veterinary anatomy and radiology which have direct bearing upon the compilation of this atlas.

We intentionally have forgone the index. It only would be a repetition of the termini technici. On the other hand, basic anatomic knowledge is a prerequisite in using the atlas for specific radiologic problems.

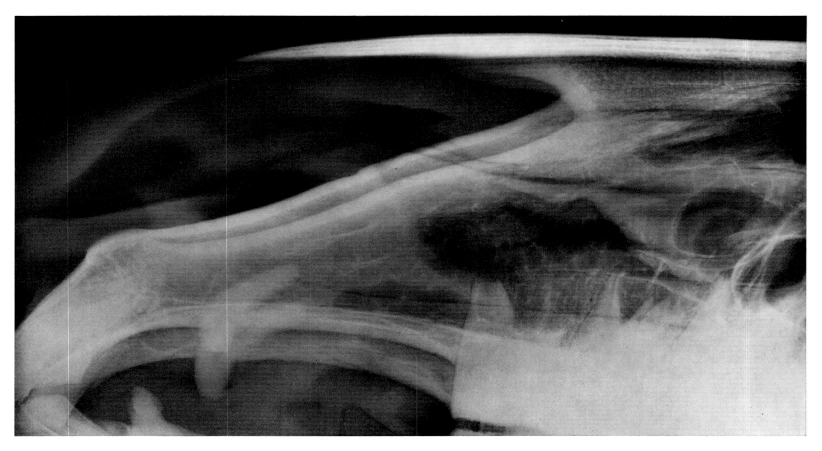

Abb. 1   Nasenhöhle (rostral). Latero-lateral. Warmblut, 12 Jahre.
Feinzeichnende Folie — FFA 120 cm — 70 kV — 30 mAs
Verkleinerung von 24 × 30 cm
Lagerung Abb. 2

Fig. 1   Nasal cavity (rostral). Laterolateral. Light horse, 12 years old.
High definition screens — FFD 120 cm — 70 kV — 30 mAs
Diminution of 24 × 30 cm
Positioning fig. 2

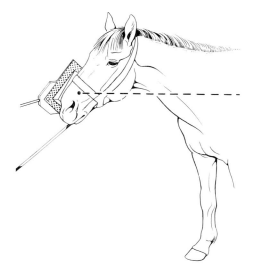

Abb. 2   Lagerung zur Aufnahme des Kopfes (rostraler Bereich). Latero-
lateral.

Die Kassette ist parallel zur Medianebene des Kopfes (oberer Kassettenrand parallel zur palpierbaren Naht zwischen den Nasenbeinen) zu lagern. Der erforderliche Abstand zwischen der rostral liegenden Kassettenkante und dem Gesicht läßt sich mit Hilfe eines Schaumgummikeils herstellen und einhalten.
Zur Aufnahme des rostralen Teiles des Gesichtsschädels (Abb. 1) sollte der
Zentralstrahl den Kopf in halber Höhe zwischen Nasenrücken und Lippenwinkel etwa ein- bis zweifingerbreit rostral des Dens praemolaris II
treffen und im rechten Winkel auf die Kassette einfallen.
Zur Aufnahme des rostralen Abschnitts des Unterkiefers (Abb. 10) sollte
der Zentralstrahl den Margo interalveolaris des Unterkiefers etwa ein-
bis zweifingerbreit rostral des Dens praemolaris II treffen und im rechten
Winkel auf die Kassette einfallen.

Fig. 2   Positioning of head (rostral part). Laterolateral.

The cassette should be placed parallel to the median plane of the head
(the upper edge of the cassette parallel to the palpable internasal suture).
The required distance between the rostral border of the cassette and
the face can be kept constant with the help of a foam rubber pad.
To obtain a radiograph of the rostral part of the face (fig. 1), the central
beam should strike the head half-way between the dorsum nasi and the
angle of the mouth, approximately one to two fingerwidths rostrally to
the 2nd premolar and fall at right angles to the cassette.
In radiographing the rostral part of the mandible (fig. 10), the central
beam should strike the interalveolar margin of the mandible approximately one to two fingerwidths rostrally to the 2nd premolar and fall
at right angles to the cassette.

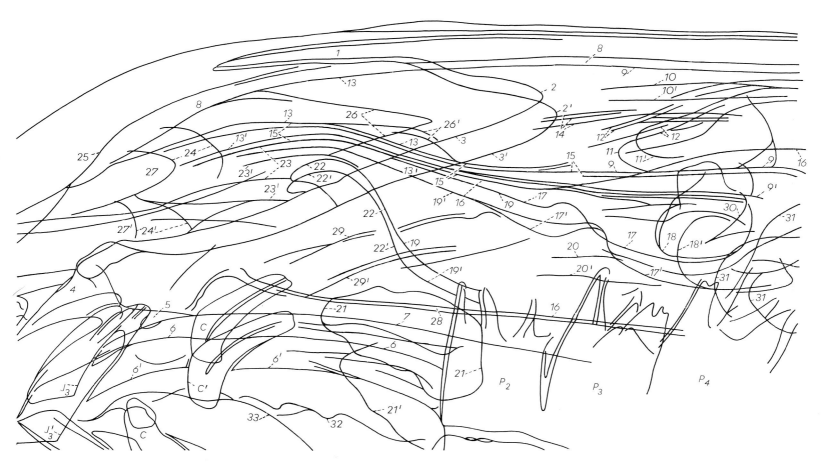

Abb. 3* Röntgenskizze zu Abb. 1   Fig. 3* X-ray sketch to fig. 1

J_3 Dens incisivus III;
C   Dens caninus;
P_2 Dens praemolaris II;
P_3 Dens praemolaris III;
P_4 Dens praemolaris IV;

Am Schädel — On the skull:

1   Os nasale, rostrales Ende — Os nasale, rostral end;
2   Incisura nasoincisiva;
3—5 Os incisivum:
3   Processus nasalis,
4   Corpus,
5   Processus palatinus;
6   Margo interalveolaris;
7   Palatum durum;
8   Meatus nasi dorsalis;
9—12 Concha nasalis dorsalis:
10   Crista ethmoidalis,
11   Bulla conchalis,
12   Orthograph getroffene Abschnitte der Spirallamellen — Orthographically struck parts of the spiral lamellae;
13   Plica recta;

14   Aufhellung, die sich aus der Aufteilung der Plica recta in einen dorsalen und einen ventralen Schenkel ergibt — Rarefaction formed by the division of the straight fold into a dorsal and a ventral branch;
15   Meatus nasi medius;
16—19 Concha nasalis ventralis:
17   Spirallamelle,
18   Bulla conchalis,
19   Pars rostralis, Begrenzung — Pars rostralis, limit;
20   Crista conchalis;
21   Lufthaltige Bucht im rostrodorsalen Bereich des Backenvorhofs — Air-containing recess in the rostrodorsal region of buccal vestible;
22   Cartilago nasalis accessoria medialis;
23   Plica alaris;
24   Cartilago alaris;
25   Cartilago nasi lateralis dorsalis;
26   Diverticulum nasi;
27   Naris;
28   Meatus nasi ventralis;
29   Canalis alveolaris;
30   Foramen infraorbitale;
31   Sinus maxillaris rostralis, rostrale Begrenzung — Sinus maxillaris rostralis, rostral limit;
32   Ruga palatina;
33   Apex linguae.

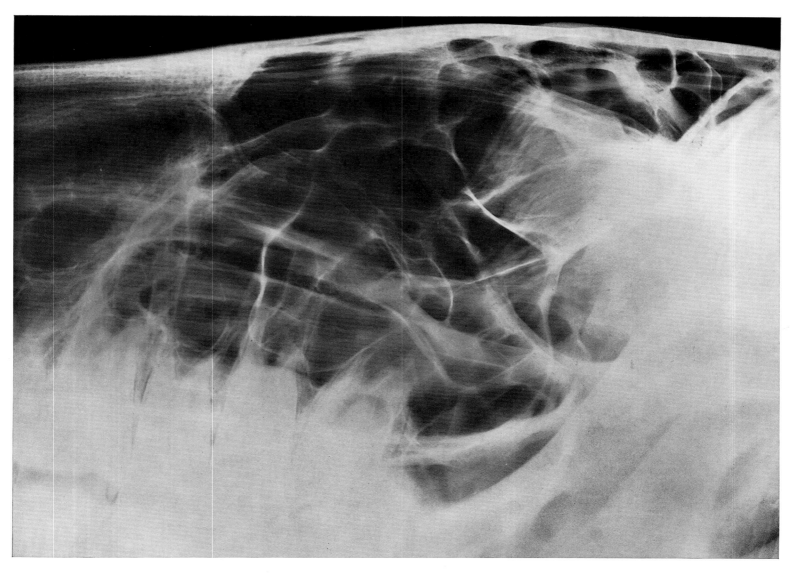

Abb. 4   Nasennebenhöhlen. Latero-lateral. Warmblut, 12 Jahre.
Feinzeichnende Folie — FFA 120 cm — 65 kV — 60 mAs
Verkleinerung von 24 × 30 cm
Lagerung Abb. 5

Fig. 4   Paranasal sinuses. Laterolateral. Light horse, 12 years old.
High definition screens — FFD 120 cm — 65 kV — 60 mAs
Diminution of 24 × 30 cm
Positioning fig. 5

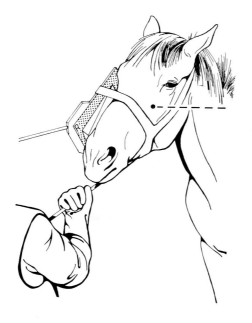

Abb. 5   Lagerung zur Aufnahme der Nasennebenhöhlen.
Latero-lateral.
Die Kassette ist parallel zur Medianebene (oberer Kassettenrand parallel
zur palpierbaren Naht zwischen den Nasenbeinen) zu lagern. Der erforderliche Abstand zwischen der rostral liegenden Kassettenkante und
dem Gesicht läßt sich mit Hilfe eines Schaumgummikeils herstellen und
einhalten.
Der Zentralstrahl sollte zweifingerbreit dorsal und zweifingerbreit kaudal des rostralen Endes der Crista facialis den Kopf treffen und im rechten Winkel auf die Kassette einfallen.

Fig. 5   Positioning of paranasal sinuses. Laterolateral.
The cassette should be placed parallel to the median plane (the upper
edge of the cassette parallel to the palpable internasal suture). The required distance between the rostral border of the cassette and the face
can be kept constant with the help of a foam rubber pad.
The central beam should strike the head two fingerwidths dorsally and
two fingerwidths caudally from the rostral end of the facial crest and
fall at right angles to the cassette.

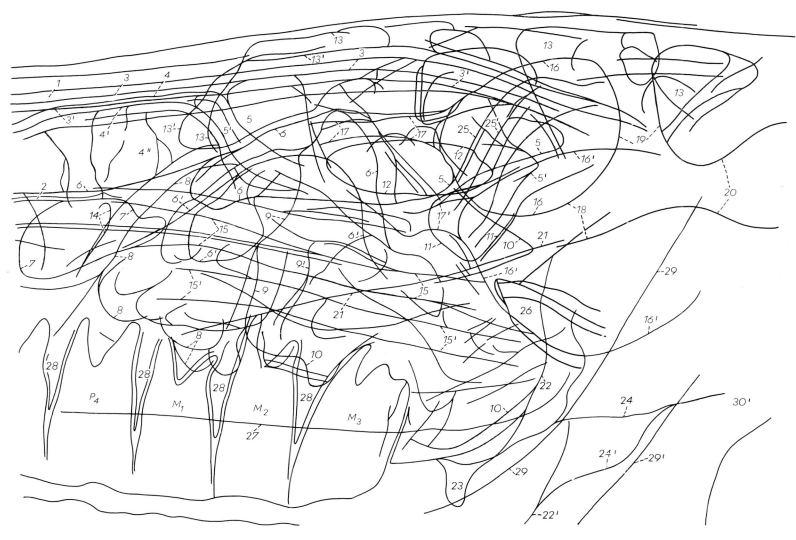

Abb. 6* Röntgenskizze zu Abb. 4   Fig. 6* X-ray sketch to fig. 4

P₄ Dens praemolaris IV;
M₁ Dens molaris I;
M₂ Dens molaris II;
M₃ Dens molaris III;

Am Schädel — On the skull:

1   Meatus nasi dorsalis;
2   Meatus nasi medius;
3—5 Concha nasalis dorsalis:
3   Dorsale Begrenzung — Dorsal limit,
4   Pars rostralis et Bulla conchalis (4″),
5   Sinus conchae dorsalis, Begrenzung abschnittsweise dargestellt —
    Sinus conchae dorsalis, partially delimited;
6, 7 Concha nasalis ventralis:
6   Dorsale Begrenzung abschnittsweise dargestellt — Dorsal limit partly
    shown,
7   Bulla conchalis partis rostralis;
8   Sinus maxillaris rostralis;
9   Septum sinuum maxillarium;
10 Sinus maxillaris caudalis;

11 Concha nasalis media et Sinus conchae mediae;
12 Apertura frontomaxillaris;
13 Sinus frontalis;
14 Foramen infraorbitale;
15 Canalis infraorbitalis;
16 Orbita;
17 Canalis lacrimalis;
18 Os zygomaticum, Processus temporalis;
19 Os frontale, Processus zygomaticus;
20 Os temporale, Processus zygomaticus;
21 Crista facialis;
22 Tuber maxillae;
23 Hamulus pterygoideus;
24 Processus pterygoideus;
25 Os ethmoidale;
26 Sinus palatinus;
27 Palatum durum;
28 Septum interalveolarium;
29 Ramus mandibulae;
30 Processus coronoideus.

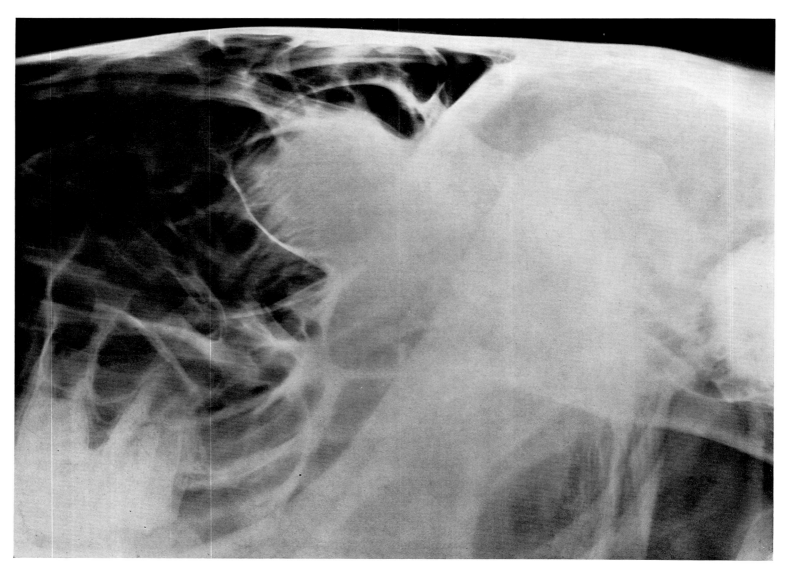

Abb. 7 Nasennebenhöhlen, kaudaler Bereich. Latero-lateral. Warmblut, 12 Jahre.
Feinzeichnende Folie — FFA 120 cm — 70 kV — 50 mAs
Verkleinerung von 24 × 30 cm
Lagerung Abb. 8

Fig. 7 Paranasal sinuses, caudal part. Laterolateral. Light horse, 12 years old.
High definition screens — FFD 120 cm — 70 kV — 50 mAs
Diminution of 24 × 30 cm
Positioning fig. 8

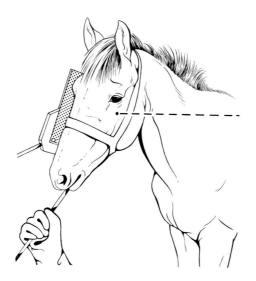

Abb. 8 Lagerung zur Aufnahme der Nasennebenhöhlen, kaudaler
Bereich. Latero-lateral.

Die Kassette ist dem Kopf so anzulegen, daß der rostrale Kassettenrand dem Lippenwinkel, der kaudale Kassettenrand der Crista facialis anliegt. Der Zentralstrahl sollte den Kopf zweifingerbreit rostral und zweifingerbreit ventral des temporalen Lidwinkels treffen und im rechten Winkel auf die Kassette einfallen. Durch die relativ geringe Schräglagerung werden der Bereich der Fossa pterygopalatina und die Gaumenhöhle besser dargestellt.

Fig. 8 Positioning of paranasal sinuses, caudal part. Laterolateral.

The cassette should be placed against the head in such a manner that the rostral end contacts the angle of the mouth and the caudal end the facial crest.
The central beam should strike the head at a point two fingerwidths rostrally and just as far ventrally from the lateral commissure of the eyelid and fall at right angles to the cassette. The region of the pterygopalatine fossa and the palatine sinus can be depicted better by this relatively slight oblique positioning.

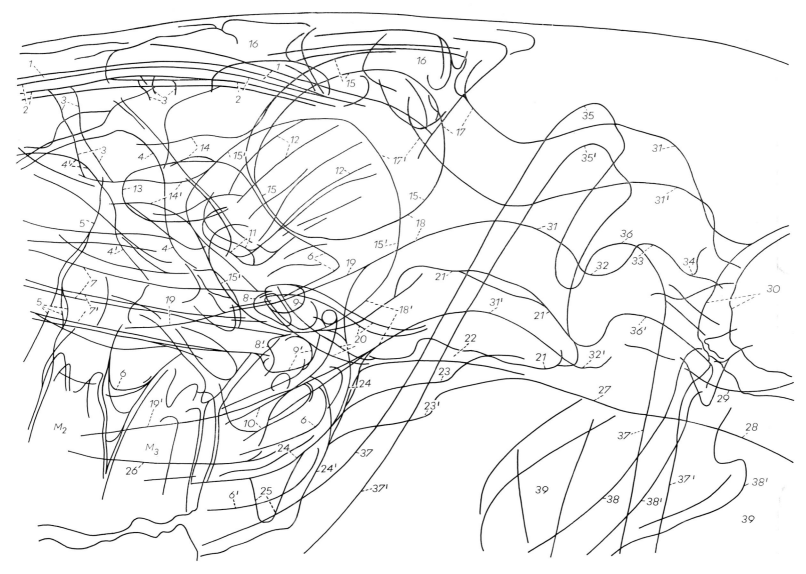

Abb. 9* Röntgenskizze zu Abb. 7   Fig. 9* X-ray sketch to fig. 7

M₂ Dens molaris II;
M₃ Dens molaris III;

Am Schädel — On the skull:

1 Meatus nasi dorsalis;
2 Concha nasalis dorsalis, dorsale Begrenzung — Concha nasalis dorsalis, dorsal limit;
3 Sinus conchae dorsalis, Knochenleisten in der medialen Wand — Sinus conchae dorsalis, bone ridges in the medial wall;
4 Concha nasalis ventralis, kaudale Begrenzung — Concha nasalis ventralis, caudal limit;
5 Septum sinuum maxillarium;
6 Sinus maxillaris caudalis;
7 Canalis infraorbitalis;
8 Foramen maxillare;
9 Foramen sphenopalatinum;
10 Canalis palatinus;
11 Concha nasalis media et Sinus conchae mediae;
12 Ethmoturbinalia;
13 Apertura frontomaxillaris;
14 Canalis lacrimalis;
15 Orbita;
16 Sinus frontalis;

17 Os frontale, Processus zygomaticus;
18 Os zygomaticum, Processus temporalis;
19 Crista facialis;
20 Sinus palatinus;
21 Sinus sphenoidalis;
22 Os praesphenoidale;
23 Processus pterygoideus;
24 Tuber maxillae;
25 Hamulus pterygoideus;
26 Palatum durum;
27 Os basisphenoidale;
28 Os occipitale, Pars basilaris;
29 Foramen lacerum;
30 Felsenbeinpyramide — Petrous temporal bone;
31 Os temporale, Processus zygomaticus;
32 Tuberculum articulare;
33 Fossa mandibularis;
34 Processus retroarticularis;
35 Processus coronoideus;
36 Processus condylaris;
37 Ramus mandibulae;
38 Os hyoideum;
39 Diverticulum tubae auditivae.

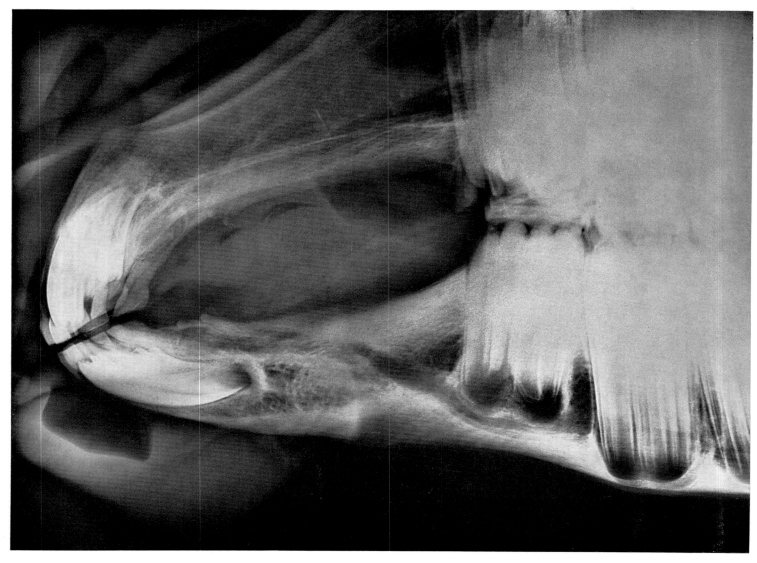

Abb. 10   Mundhöhle, rostraler Bereich. Latero-lateral. Warmblut, 2¹/₂ Jahre.
Feinzeichnende Folie — FFA 100 cm — 55 kV — 52 mAs
Verkleinerung von 24 × 30 cm
Lagerung Abb. 2

Fig. 10   Oral cavity, rostral part. Laterolateral. Light horse, 2¹/₂ years old.
High definition screens — FFD 100 cm — 55 kV — 52 mAs
Diminution of 24 × 30 cm
Positioning fig. 2

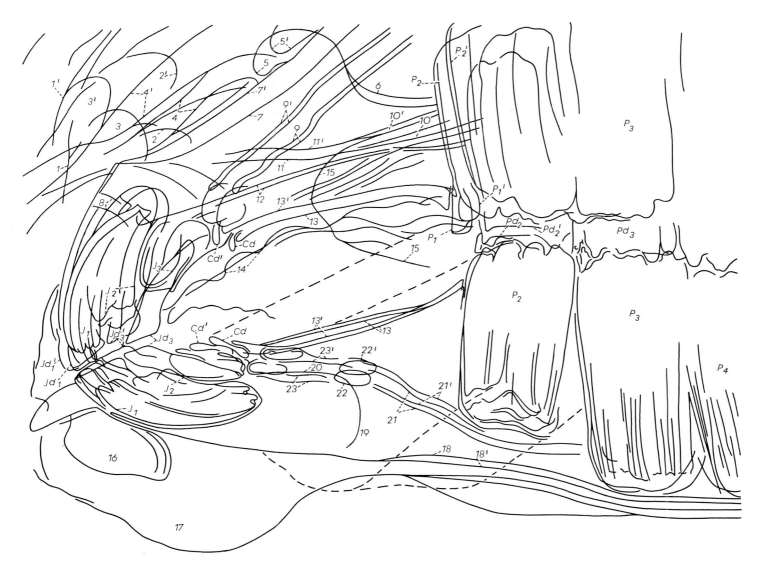

Abb. 11* Röntgenskizze zu Abb. 10
Gestrichelte Linie: Strickhalfter

Fig. 11* X-ray sketch to Fig. 10
Broken line: cord halter

Dentes decidui:

Jd₁ Dens incisivus deciduus I;
Jd₃ Dens incisivus deciduus III;
Cd Dens caninus deciduus;
Pd₂ Dens praemolaris deciduus II;
Pd₃ Dens praemolaris deciduus III;

Dentes permanentes:

J₁ Dens incisivus I, Anlage — 1st incisor tooth, primordium;
J₂ Dens incisivus II, Anlage — 2nd incisor tooth, primordium;
J₃ Dens incisivus III, Anlage — 3rd incisor tooth, primordium;
P₁ Dens praemolaris I;
P₂ Dens praemolaris II;
P₃ Dens praemolaris III;
P₄ Dens praemolaris IV;

Am Cranium — On the cranium:

1, 2 Cartilago alaris:
1 Cornu,
2 Lamina;
3 Naris;
4 Plica alaris;

5 Cartilago nasalis accessoria medialis;
6 Bulla conchalis partis rostralis conchae nasalis ventralis;
7 Os incisivum, Processus nasalis;
8 Canalis interincisivus;
9 Canalis alveolaris;
10 Meatus nasi ventralis;
11 Plica basalis;
12 Os incisivum, Processus palatinus;
13 Margo interalveolaris;
14 Ruga palatina;
15 Lufthaltige Bucht im rostrodorsalen Bereich des Backenvorhofs — Air-containing recess in the rostrodorsal region of buccal vestible;

An der Mandibula — On the mandible:

16 Vestibulum labiale;
17 Mentum;
18 Corpus mandibulae;
19 Kinnwinkel — Angle of chin;
20 Verschattung, die sich aus der Konkavität der Pars incisiva ergibt — Shadow formed by the concavity of pars incisiva;
21 Canalis mandibulae;
22 Foramen mentale;
23 Canalis alveolaris.

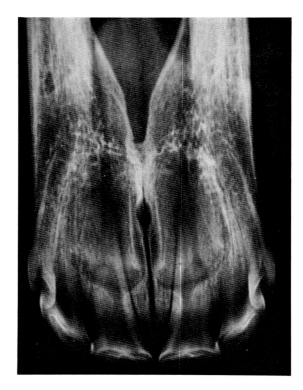

Abb. 12 Oberkieferschneidezähne (Kassette in die Mundhöhle einge-
legt). Schrägprojektion. Dorso-ventral. Vollblut, 1 Jahr.
Feinzeichnende Folie — FFA 100 cm — 40 kV — 10 mAs
Originalgröße
Lagerung Abb. 14

Fig. 12 Maxillary incisor teeth (cassette placed in oral cavity).
Obliquely dorsoventral. Thoroughbred, 1 year old.
High definition screens — FFD 100 cm — 40 kV — 10 mAs
Original size
Positioning fig. 14

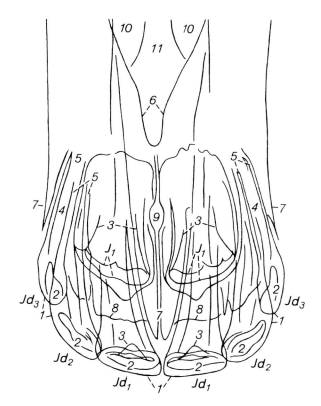

Abb. 13 Röntgenskizze zu Abb. 12

Fig. 13 X-ray sketch to fig. 12

Dentes decidui:
Jd₁ Dens incisivus deciduus I;
Jd₂ Dens incisivus deciduus II;
Jd₃ Dens incisivus deciduus III;

Dens permanens:
J₁ Dens incisivus I, Anlage — 1st incisor tooth, primordium;

An den Zähnen — On the teeth:
1 Corona dentis;
2 Facies occlusalis;
3 Infundibulum dentis;
4 Cavum dentis;
5 Canalis radicis dentis et Foramen apicis dentis;

Am Cranium — On the cranium:
6 Winkel zwischen den Processus nasales der Ossa incisiva — Angle
between the nasal processes of the incisive bones;
7 Alveolus dentalis;
8 Margo alveolaris, abschnittsweise dargestellt — Margo alveolaris,
only partly shown;
9 Canalis incisivus;
10 Fissura palatina;
11 Septum nasi.

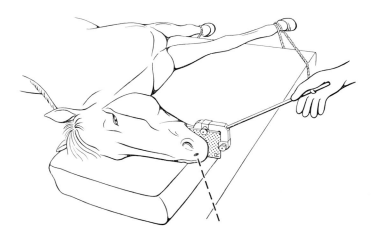

Abb. 14 Lagerung zur Aufnahme der Oberkieferschneidezähne.
Schrägprojektion. Dorso-ventral.

Die Mundspalte ist nach dem Einlegen der Kassette — bei Fohlen und
Shetlandponys nach Einlegen des folienlosen Filmes und des Bleilatzes —
vorsichtig zu schließen.
Bei der Einstellung des Zentralstrahls ist darauf zu achten, daß keine
seitliche Verkantung entsteht.
Der Zentralstrahl sollte bei bis zu 10 Jahre alten Pferden im Winkel von
ca. 25° und bei älteren Tieren im Winkel von ca. 20° auf den Film einfallen.

Fig. 14 Positioning of maxillary incisor teeth.
Obliquely dorsoventral.

After inserting the cassette the mouth should be closed carefully. In foals
and Shetland ponys a non-screen film and lead shielding should be
employed.
During alignment of the central beam care should be taken to avoid
sideways tilting.
In horses up to 10 years of age the central beam should strike the film
at an angle of 25° and in older animals at an angle of 20°.

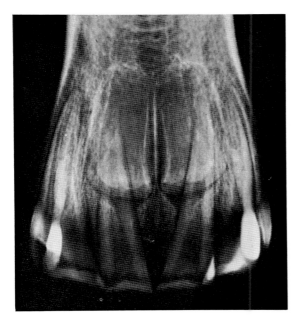

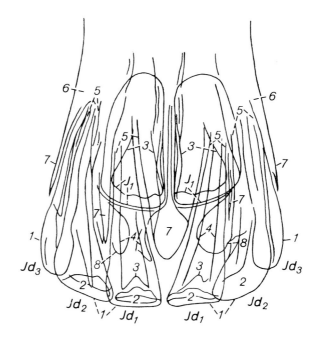

Abb. 15 Unterkieferschneidezähne (Kassette in die Mundhöhle eingelegt). Schrägprojektion. Ventro-dorsal. Vollblut, 1 Jahr.
Feinzeichnende Folie — FFA 100 cm — 42 kV — 7 mAs
Originalgröße
Lagerung Abb. 17

Fig. 15 Mandibular incisor teeth (cassette placed in oral cavity). Obliquely ventrodorsal. Thoroughbred, 1 year old.
High definition screens — FFD 100 cm — 42 kV — 7 mAs
Original size
Positioning fig. 17

Abb. 16 Röntgenskizze zu Abb. 15

Fig. 16 X-ray sketch to fig. 15

Dentes decidui:
Jd₁ Dens incisivus deciduus I;
Jd₂ Dens incisivus deciduus II;
Jd₃ Dens incisivus deciduus III;

Dens permanens:
J₁ Dens incisivus I, Anlage — 1st incisor tooth, primordium;

An den Zähnen — On the teeth:

1 Corona dentis;
2 Facies occlusalis;
3 Infundibulum dentis;
4 Cavum dentis;
5 Canalis radicis dentis et Foramen apicis dentis;

An der Mandibula — On the mandible:

6 Pars incisiva mandibulae;
7 Alveolus dentalis;
8 Margo alveolaris, abschnittsweise dargestellt — Margo alveolaris, only partly shown.

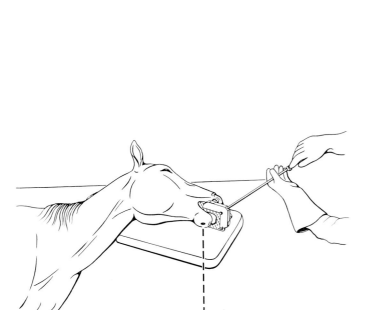

Abb. 17 Lagerung zur Aufnahme der Unterkieferschneidezähne.
Schrägprojektion. Ventro-dorsal.

Die Mundspalte ist nach dem Einlegen der Kassette — bei Fohlen und Shetlandponys nach Einlegen des folienlosen Filmes und des Bleilatzes — vorsichtig zu schließen.
Bei der Einstellung des Zentralstrahls ist darauf zu achten, daß keine seitliche Verkantung entsteht.
Der Zentralstrahl sollte bei bis zu 10 Jahre alten Pferden im Winkel von ca. 20° und bei älteren Tieren im Winkel von ca. 15° auf den Film einfallen.

Fig. 17 Positioning of mandibular incisor teeth.
Obliquely ventrodorsal.

After inserting the cassette the mouth should be closed carefully. In foals and Shetland ponys a non-screen film and lead shielding should be employed.
During alignment of the central beam care should be taken to avoid sideways tilting.
In horses up to 10 years of age the central beam should strike the film at an angle of 20° and in older animals at an angle of 15°.

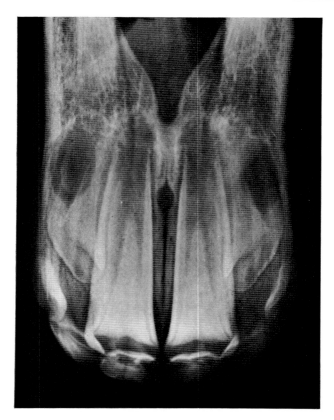

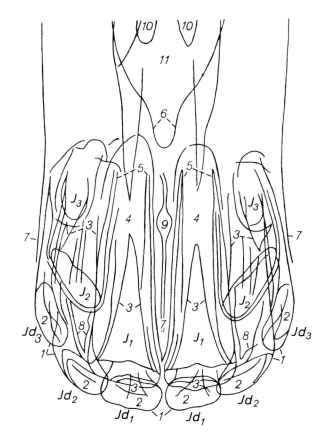

Abb. 18 Oberkieferschneidezähne (Kassette in die Mundhöhle einge-
legt). Schrägprojektion. Dorso-ventral. Warmblut, 2 Jahre.
Feinzeichnende Folie — FFA 100 cm — 50 kV — 12 mAs
Originalgröße
Lagerung Abb. 14

Fig. 18 Maxillary incisor teeth (cassette placed in oral cavity).
Obliquely dorsoventral. Light horse, 2 years old.
High definition screens — FFD 100 cm — 50 kV — 12 mAs
Original size
Positioning fig. 14

Abb. 19 Röntgenskizze zu Abb. 18
(Legende s. S. 21)

Fig. 19 X-ray sketch to fig. 18
(Legend see p. 21)

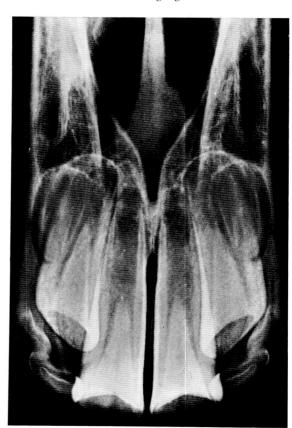

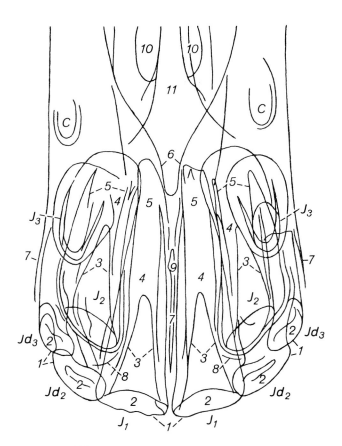

Abb. 20 Oberkieferschneidezähne (Kassette in die Mundhöhle einge-
legt). Schrägprojektion. Dorso-ventral. Traber, 3 Jahre.
Feinzeichnende Folie — FFA 100 cm — 45 kV — 8 mAs
Originalgröße
Lagerung Abb. 14

Fig. 20 Maxillary incisor teeth (cassette placed in oral cavity).
Obliquely dorsoventral. Trotter, 3 years old.
High definition screens — FFD 100 cm — 45 kV — 8 mAs
Original size
Positioning fig. 14

Abb. 21 Röntgenskizze zu Abb. 20
(Legende s. S. 21)

Fig. 21 X-ray sketch to fig. 20
(Legend see p. 21)

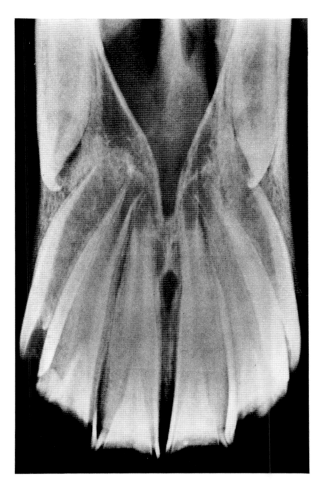

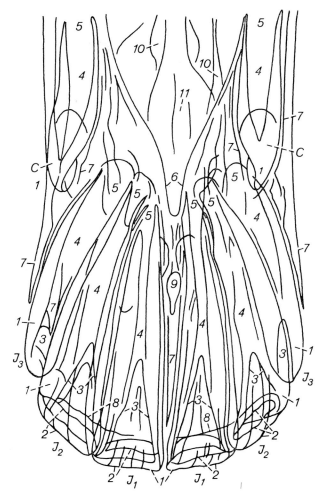

Abb. 22 Oberkieferschneidezähne (Kassette in die Mundhöhle einge-
legt). Schrägprojektion. Dorso-ventral. Traber ♂, 5 Jahre.
Feinzeichnende Folie — FFA 100 cm — 50 kV — 7 mAs
Originalgröße
Lagerung Abb. 14

Fig. 22 Maxillary incisor teeth (cassette placed in oral cavity).
Obliquely dorsoventral. Trotter ♂, 5 years old.
High definition screens — FFD 100 cm — 50 kV — 7 mAs
Original size
Positioning fig. 14

Abb. 23 Röntgenskizze zu Abb. 22

Fig. 23 X-ray sketch to fig. 22

Legende zu Abb. 19 — Legend to fig. 19

Dentes decidui:

Jd_1 Dens incisivus deciduus I;
Jd_2 Dens incisivus deciduus II;
Jd_3 Dens incisivus deciduus III;

Dentes permanentes:

J_1 Dens incisivus I, Anlage — 1st incisor tooth, primordium;
J_2 Dens incisivus II, Anlage — 2nd incisor tooth, primordium;
J_3 Dens incisivus III, Anlage — 3rd incisor tooth, primordium;

Legende zu Abb. 21 — Legend to fig. 21

Dentes decidui:

Jd_2 Dens incisivus deciduus II;
Jd_3 Dens incisivus deciduus III;

Dentes permanentes:

J_1 Dens incisivus I;
J_2 Dens incisivus II, Anlage — 2nd incisor tooth, primordium;
J_3 Dens incisivus III, Anlage — 3rd incisor tooth, primordium;
C Dens caninus, Anlage — Canine tooth, primordium;

Legende zu Abb. 23 — Legend to fig. 23

Dentes permanentes:

J_1 Dens incisivus I;
J_2 Dens incisivus II;
J_3 Dens incisivus III;
C Dens caninus;

**Gemeinsame Legende zu den Abb. 19, 21, 23 —
Common legend to figs. 19, 21, 23**

An den Zähnen — On the teeth:

1 Corona dentis;
2 Facies occlusalis;
3 Infundibulum dentis;
4 Cavum dentis;
5 Canalis radicis dentis et Foramen apicis dentis;

Am Cranium — On the cranium:

6 Winkel zwischen den Processus nasales der Ossa incisiva — Angle between the nasal processes of the incisive bones;
7 Alveolus dentalis;
8 Margo alveolaris, abschnittsweise dargestellt — Margo alveolaris, only partly shown;
9 Canalis incisivus;
10 Fissura palatina;
11 Septum nasi.

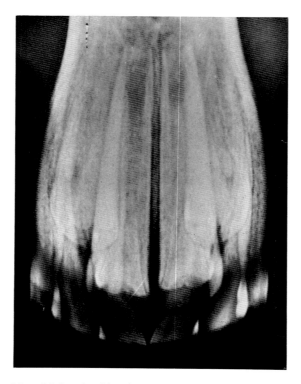

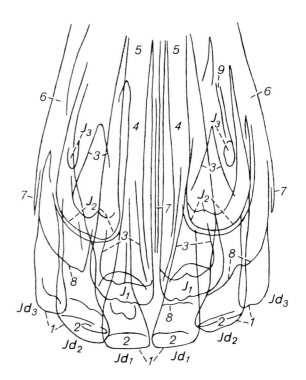

Abb. 24 Unterkieferschneidezähne (Kassette in die Mundhöhle ein-
gelegt). Schrägprojektion. Ventro-dorsal. Warmblut, 2 Jahre.
Feinzeichnende Folie — FFA 100 cm — 45 kV — 8 mAs
Originalgröße
Lagerung Abb. 17

Fig. 24 Mandibular incisor teeth (cassette placed in oral cavity).
Obliquely ventrodorsal. Light horse, 2 years old.
High definition screens — FFD 100 cm — 45 kV — 8 mAs
Original size
Positioning fig. 17

Abb. 25 Röntgenskizze zu Abb. 24
(Legende s. S. 23)

Fig. 25 X-ray sketch to fig. 24
(Legend see p. 23)

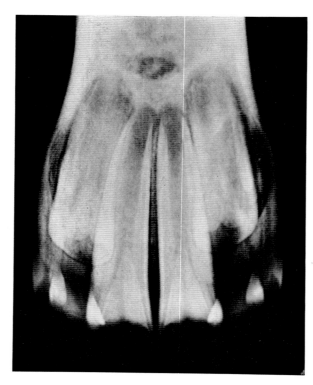

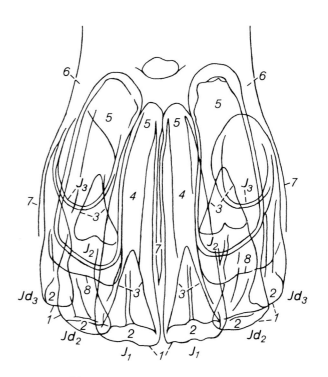

Abb. 26 Unterkieferschneidezähne (Kassette in die Mundhöhle ein-
gelegt). Schrägprojektion. Ventro-dorsal. Traber, 3 Jahre.
Feinzeichnende Folie — FFA 100 cm — 42 kV — 7 mAs
Originalgröße
Lagerung Abb. 17

Fig. 26 Mandibular incisor teeth (cassette placed in oral cavity).
Obliquely ventrodorsal. Trotter, 3 years old.
High definition screens — FFD 100 cm — 42 kV — 7 mAs
Original size
Positioning fig. 17

Abb. 27 Röntgenskizze zu Abb. 26
(Legende s. S. 23)

Fig. 27 X-ray sketch to fig. 26
(Legend see p. 23)

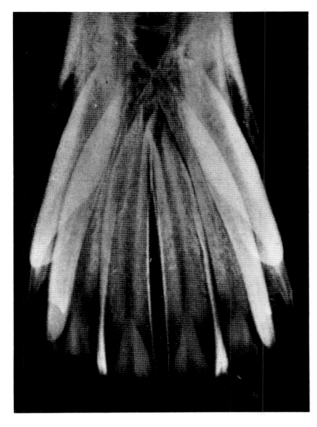

Abb. 28 Unterkieferschneidezähne (Kassette in die Mundhöhle ein-
gelegt). Schrägprojektion. Ventro-dorsal. Traber ♂, 5 Jahre.
Feinzeichnende Folie — FFA 100 cm — 46 kV — 8 mAs
Originalgröße
Lagerung Abb. 17

Fig. 28 Mandibular incisor teeth (cassette placed in oral cavity).
Obliquely ventrodorsal. Trotter ♂, 5 years old.
High definition screens — FFD 100 cm — 46 kV — 8 mAs
Original size
Positioning fig. 17

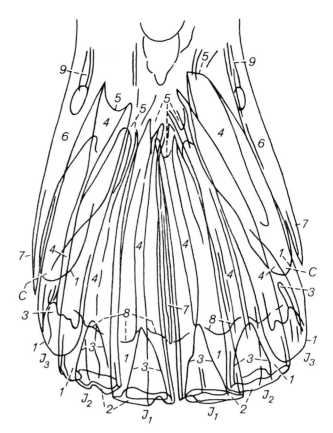

Abb. 29 Röntgenskizze zu Abb. 28

Fig. 29 X-ray sketch to fig. 28

Legende zu Abb. 25 — Legend to fig. 25

Dentes decidui:

Jd₁ Dens incisivus deciduus I;
Jd₂ Dens incisivus deciduus II;
Jd₃ Dens incisivus deciduus III;

Dentes permanentes:

J₁ Dens incisivus I, Anlage — 1st incisor tooth, primordium;
J₂ Dens incisivus II, Anlage — 2nd incisor tooth, primordium;
J₃ Dens incisivus III, Anlage — 3rd incisor tooth, primordium;

Legende zu Abb. 27 — Legend to fig. 27

Dentes decidui:

Jd₂ Dens incisivus deciduus II;
Jd₃ Dens incisivus deciduus III;

Dentes permanentes:

J₁ Dens incisivus I;
J₂ Dens incisivus II, Anlage — 2nd incisor tooth, primordium;
J₃ Dens incisivus III, Anlage — 3rd incisor tooth, primordium;

Legende zu Abb. 29 — Legend to fig. 29

Dentes permanentes:

J₁ Dens incisivus I;
J₂ Dens incisivus II;
J₃ Dens incisivus III;
C Dens caninus;

Gemeinsame Legende zu den Abb. 25, 27, 29 —
Common legend to figs. 25, 27, 29

An den Zähnen — On the teeth:

1 Corona dentis;
2 Facies occlusalis;
3 Infundibulum dentis;
4 Cavum dentis;
5 Canalis radicis dentis et Foramen apicis dentis;

An der Mandibula — On the mandible:

6 Pars incisiva mandibulae;
7 Alveolus dentalis;
8 Margo alveolaris, abschnittsweise dargestellt — Margo alveolaris,
only partly shown;
9 Canalis alveolaris.

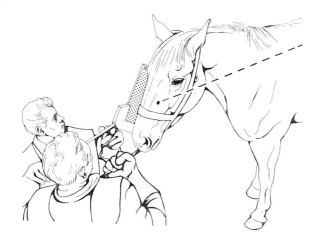

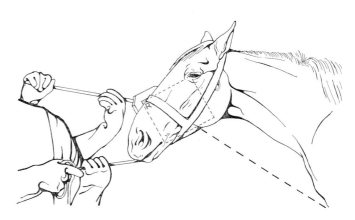

Abb. 30 Lagerung zur Aufnahme der maxillaren Backenzähne. Schrägprojektion. Latero-lateral.

Die Kassette ist parallel zur Medianebene des Kopfes (obere Kassettenkante parallel zur palpierbaren Naht zwischen den Nasenbeinen) zu lagern. Die obere Kassettenkante sollte etwa 2 cm oberhalb des Nasenrückens, die rostral liegende Kassettenkante etwa fingerbreit vor dem ersten Backenzahn liegen. Der erforderliche Abstand zwischen der rostral liegenden Kassettenkante und dem Kopf läßt sich mit Hilfe eines Schaumgummikeils herstellen und einhalten.

Der Zentralstrahl sollte den Kopf in einem Winkel von 25° von oben her 2—3 fingerbreit dorsal des rostralen Endes der Crista facialis treffen.

Fig. 30 Positioning of maxillary cheek teeth. Obliquely laterolateral.

The cassette should be placed parallel to the median plane of the head (the upper edge of the cassette parallel to the palpable internasal suture). The upper edge of the cassette should rest approximately 2 cm dorsal to the dorsum nasi and the rostral edge approximately one fingerwidth rostrally to the 1st premolar. The required distance between the rostral end of the cassette and the head can be secured and kept steady with the help of a foam rubber pad.

The central beam should strike the head from above at a width of 2—3 fingers dorsally to the rostral end of the facial crest at an angle of 25°.

Abb. 31 Lagerung zur Aufnahme der mandibularen Backenzähne. Schrägprojektion. Latero-lateral.

Der Kopf des Pferdes ist gestreckt zu halten. Die Kassette liegt dem Unterkiefer an. Die rostral liegende Kassettenkante befindet sich etwa 3 cm vor dem ersten Backenzahn, ihre untere Kante etwa fingerbreit unterhalb des Unterkieferrands.

Der Zentralstrahl sollte in Höhe des rostralen Endes der Crista facialis von ventral her in einem Winkel von 45° die Mitte des Kehlgangs treffen.

Fig. 31 Positioning of mandibular cheek teeth. Obliquely laterolateral.

The head of the horse must be held in a stretched position. The cassette rests on the mandible. The rostral edge of the cassette is placed approximately 3 cm rostrally to the 1st premolar, the ventral edge approximately one fingerwidth ventral to the border of the mandible.

The central beam should strike the center of the intermandibular space from ventral at an angle of 45° on a level of the rostral end of the facial crest.

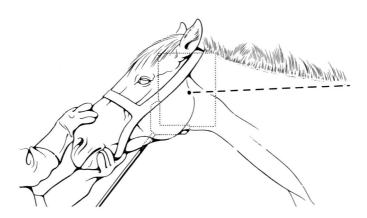

Abb. 32 Lagerung zur Aufnahme des Luftsacks. Latero-lateral.

Bei maximal nach vorn gestrecktem Kopf ist die Kassette parallel zur Medianebene (Kassettenkante parallel zur Naht zwischen den Stirn- und den Nasenbeinen) zu lagern. Die Kassette muß dem lateralen Lidwinkel und dem Ohrgrund anliegen.

Der Zentralstrahl sollte den hinteren Rand der Mandibula etwa 10 cm unterhalb des Ohrgrunds treffen und im rechten Winkel auf die Kassette einfallen.

Fig. 32 Positioning of guttural pouch. Laterolateral.

The cassette should be placed parallel to the median plane with the head in maximal extension (the edge of the cassette parallel to the suture between the frontal and nasal bones). The cassette must rest on the lateral commissure of the eyelid and the base of the external ear.

The central beam should strike the caudal border of the mandible approximately 10 cm ventrally to the base of the external ear and fall at right angles to the cassette.

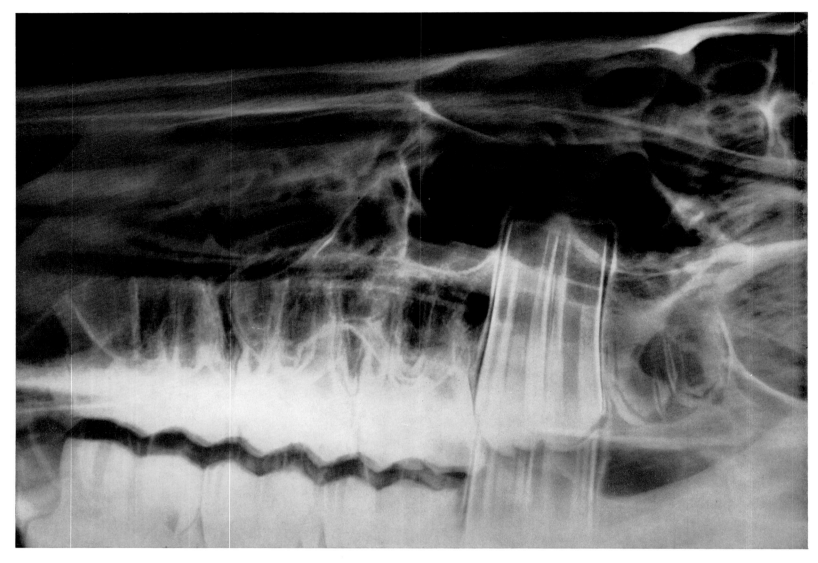

Abb. 33   Maxillare Backenzähne. Schrägprojektion. Latero-lateral. Vollblut, 1 Jahr.
Feinzeichnende Folie — FFA 90 cm — 60 kV — 50 mAs
Originalgröße (Ausschnitt aus 24 × 30 cm)
Lagerung Abb. 30

Fig. 33   Maxillary cheek teeth. Obliquely laterolateral. Thoroughbred, 1 year old.
High definition screens — FFD 90 cm — 60 kV — 50 mAs
Original size (section of 24 × 30 cm)
Positioning fig. 30

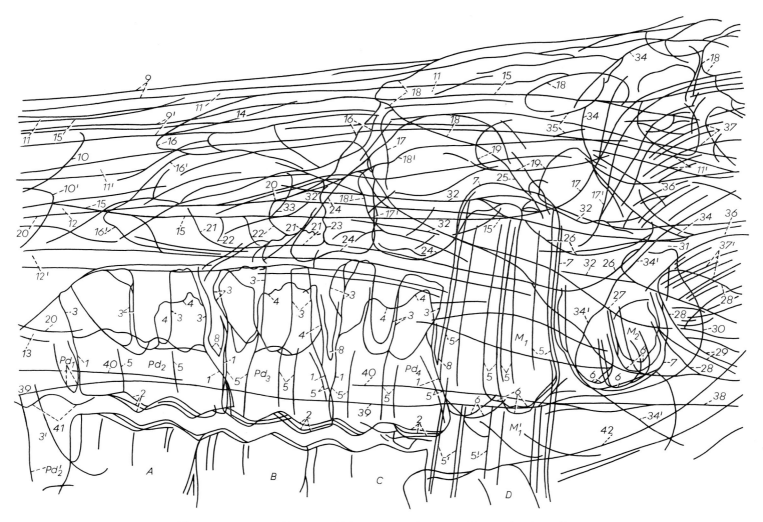

Abb. 34* Röntgenskizze zu Abb. 33   Fig. 34* X-ray sketch to fig. 33

Im Arcus dentalis maxillaris — In the maxillary dental arch:

P_1 Dens praemolaris I;
Pd_2 Dens praemolaris deciduus II;
Pd_3 Dens praemolaris deciduus III;
Pd_4 Dens praemolaris deciduus IV;
M_1 Dens molaris I;
M_2 Dens molaris II, Anlage — 2nd molar tooth, primordium;

Im Arcus dentalis mandibularis — In the mandibular dental arch:

A Dens praemolaris deciduus II;
B Dens praemolaris deciduus III;
C Dens praemolaris deciduus IV;
D Dens molaris I;

An den maxillaren Backenzähnen — On the maxillary cheek teeth:

1 Corpus dentis;
2 Facies occlusalis;
3 Bukkale Radix dentis — Buccal root;
4 Palatinale Radix dentis — Palatinal root;
5 Plicae enameli, am M_1 Verschattungen, die sich aus orthograph getroffenen Abschnitten der Schmelzbecher und aus Falten des Schmelzmantels ergeben — Plicae enameli, shadows on M_1 formed by orthographically struck parts of the infundibulae and peripheral enamel folds;
6 Facies occlusalis, Tubercula;
7 Alveolus dentalis;
8 Septum interalveolarium;

Am Schädel — On the skull:

9 Os nasale, orthograph getroffener Abschnitt des Nasendachs — Os nasale, orthographically struck part of the nasal roof;
10 Incisura nasoincisiva;
11 Meatus nasi dorsalis;
12 Meatus nasi medius;
13 Meatus nasi ventralis;
14 Crista ethmoidalis;
15 Concha nasalis dorsalis;
16 Pars rostralis conchae nasalis dorsalis;
17 Sinus conchae dorsalis, rostrale bzw. kaudale Begrenzung — Sinus conchae dorsalis, rostral and caudal limits respectively;
18 Sinus frontalis;
19 Apertura frontomaxillaris;
20 Concha nasalis ventralis;
21 Pars rostralis conchae nasalis ventralis;
22 Septen der Bulla conchalis partis rostralis conchae nasalis ventralis — Septa in the bulla conchalis partis rostralis conchae nasalis ventralis;
23 Septum conchae ventralis;
24 Sinus maxillaris rostralis, Begrenzung — Sinus maxillaris rostralis, limit;
25 Septum sinuum maxillarium;
26, 27 Sinus maxillaris caudalis:
26 Ventrolaterale Abteilung — Ventrolateral part,
27 Dorsomediale Abteilung — Dorsomedial part;
28 Sinus palatinus;
29 Os palatinum;
30 Tuber maxillae;
31 Fossa pterygopalatina;
32 Canalis infraorbitalis;
33 Foramen infraorbitale;
34 Orbita;
35 Canalis lacrimalis;
36 Os zygomaticum, Processus temporalis;
37 Ethmoturbinalia;
38 Processus pterygoideus;
39 Margo alveolaris;
40 Palatum durum;
41 Rugae palatinae;
42 Mandibula.

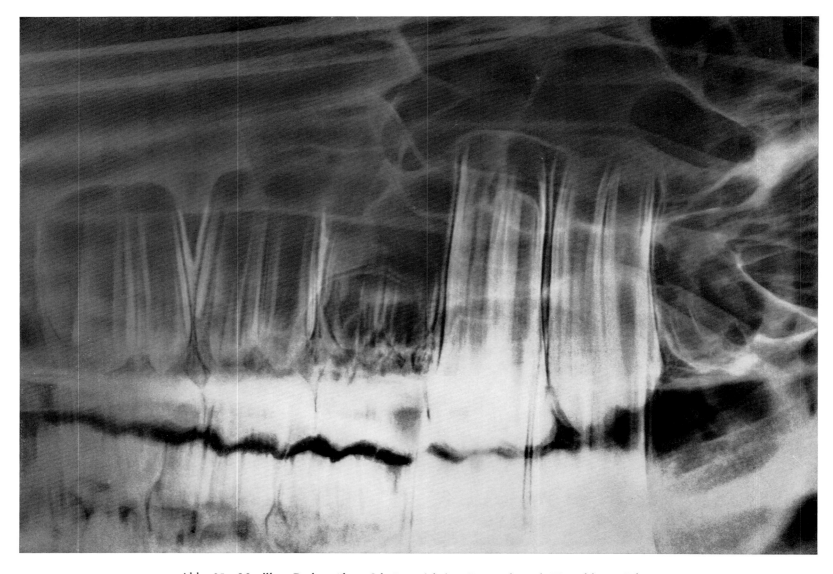

Abb. 35 Maxillare Backenzähne. Schrägprojektion. Latero-lateral. Warmblut, 2 Jahre.
Feinzeichnende Folie — FFA 120 cm — 65 kV — 55 mAs
Originalgröße (Ausschnitt aus 24 × 30 cm)
Lagerung Abb. 30

Fig. 35 Maxillary cheek teeth. Obliquely laterolateral. Light horse, 2 years old.
High definition screens — FFD 120 cm — 65 kV — 55 mAs
Original size (section of 24 × 30 cm)
Positioning fig. 30

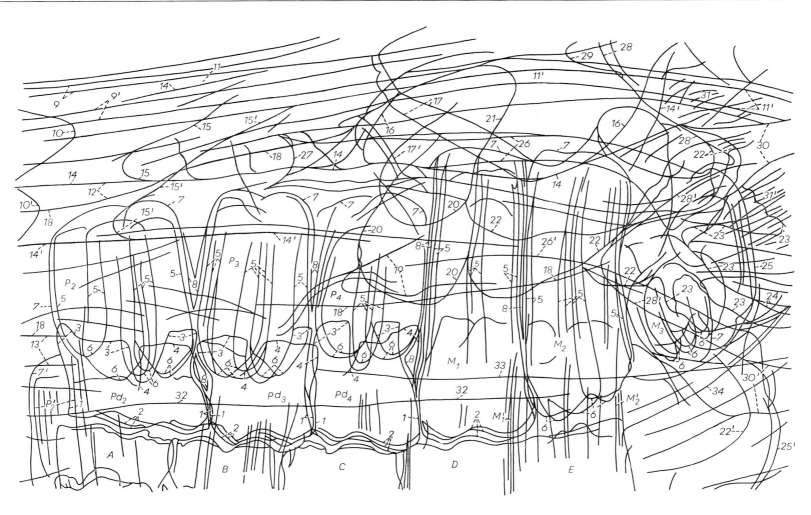

Abb. 36* Röntgenskizze zu Abb. 35   Fig. 36* X-ray sketch to fig. 35

Im Arcus dentalis maxillaris — In the maxillary dental arch:

Dentes decidui:
Pd$_2$ Dens praemolaris deciduus II;
Pd$_3$ Dens praemolaris deciduus III;
Pd$_4$ Dens praemolaris deciduus IV;

Dentes permanentes:
P$_2$ Dens praemolaris II, Anlage — 2nd premolar tooth, primordium;
P$_3$ Dens praemolaris III, Anlage — 3rd premolar tooth, primordium;
P$_4$ Dens praemolaris IV, Anlage — 4th premolar tooth, primordium;
M$_1$ Dens molaris I;
M$_2$ Dens molaris II;
M$_3$ Dens molaris III, Anlage — 3rd molar tooth, primordium;

Im Arcus dentalis mandibularis — In the mandibular dental arch:

Dentes decidui:
A   Dens praemolaris deciduus II;
B   Dens praemolaris deciduus III;
C   Dens praemolaris deciduus IV;

Dentes permanentes:
D   Dens molaris I;
E   Dens molaris II;

An den maxillaren Backenzähnen — On the maxillary cheek teeth:

1   Corpus dentis;
2   Facies occlusalis;
3   Bukkale Radix dentis — Buccal root;
4   Palatinale Radix dentis — Palatinal root;
5   Verschattungen, die sich aus orthograph getroffenen Abschnitten der Schmelzbecher und aus Plicae enameli ergeben — Shadows formed by orthographically struck parts of the infundibulae and plicae enameli;
6   Facies occlusalis, Tubercula; an der M$_3$-Anlage = Zahnscherbchen — Facies occlusalis, tubercula; parts of 3rd molar primordium;

7   Alveolus dentalis;
8   Septum interalveolarium;

Am Schädel — On the skull:

9   Os nasale, orthograph getroffener Abschnitt des Nasendachs — Os nasale, orthographically struck part of the nasal roof;
10   Incisura nasoincisiva;
11   Meatus nasi dorsalis;
12   Meatus nasi medius;
13   Meatus nasi ventralis;
14   Concha nasalis dorsalis;
15   Pars rostralis conchae nasalis dorsalis;
16   Sinus conchae dorsalis, rostrale (Septum conchae dorsalis) bzw. kaudale Begrenzung — Sinus conchae dorsalis, rostral (Septum conchae dorsalis) and caudal limits respectively;
17   Sinus frontalis, rostrale Begrenzung — Sinus frontalis, rostral limit;
18   Concha nasalis ventralis;
19   Sinus conchae ventralis;
20   Sinus maxillaris rostralis;
21   Septum sinuum maxillarium;
22   Sinus maxillaris caudalis;
23   Sinus palatinus;
24   Os palatinum;
25   Tuber maxillae;
26   Canalis infraorbitalis;
27   Foramen infraorbitale;
28   Orbita;
29   Fossa sacci lacrimalis;
30   Os zygomaticum, Processus temporalis;
31   Ethmoturbinalia;
32   Margo alveolaris;
33   Palatum durum;
34   Mandibula.

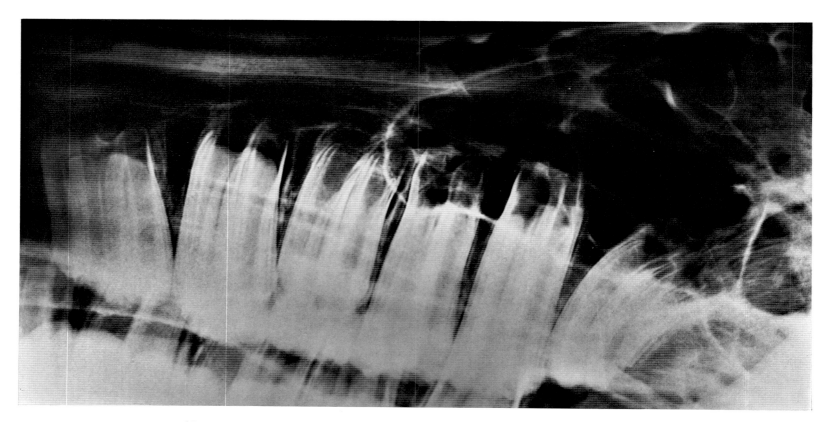

Abb. 37   Maxillare Backenzähne. Schrägprojektion. Latero-lateral. Warmblut, 3 Jahre.
Feinzeichnende Folie — FFA 100 cm — 65 kV — 30 mAs
Verkleinerung von 30 × 40 cm
Lagerung Abb. 30

Fig. 37   Maxillary cheek teeth. Obliquely laterolateral. Light horse, 3 years old.
High definition screens — FFD 100 cm — 65 kV — 30 mAs
Diminution of 30 × 40 cm
Positioning fig. 30

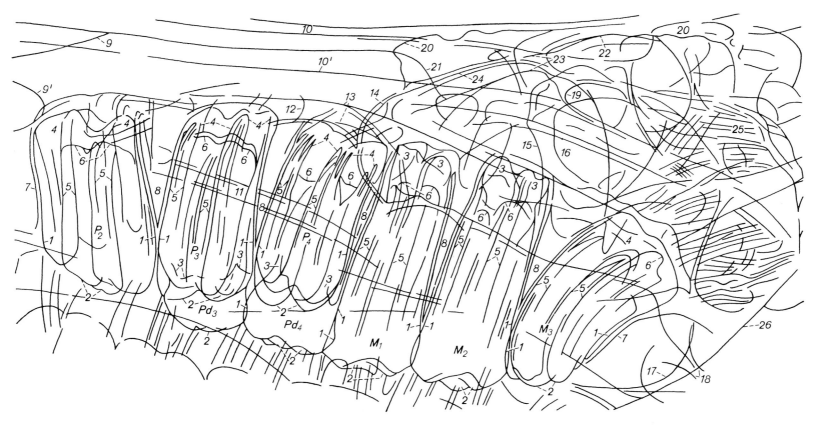

Abb. 38* Röntgenskizze zu Abb. 37   Fig. 38* X-ray sketch to fig. 37

Im Arcus dentalis maxillaris — In the maxillary dental arch:

Dentes decidui:

Pd₃ Dens praemolaris deciduus III;
Pd₄ Dens praemolaris deciduus IV;

Dentes permanentes:

P₂ Dens praemolaris II;
P₃ Dens praemolaris III, Anlage — 3rd premolar tooth, primordium;
P₄ Dens praemolaris IV, Anlage — 4th premolar tooth, primordium;
M₁ Dens molaris I;
M₂ Dens molaris II;
M₃ Dens molaris III;

An den maxillaren Backenzähnen — On the maxillary cheek teeth:

1 Corpus dentis;
2 Facies occlusalis et Tubercula coronae dentis;
3 Radices dentis,
4 Anlagen — Primordia;
5 Plicae enameli;
6 Infundibula dentis, Grund — Infundibula dentis, base;
7 Alveolus dentalis;
8 Septa interalveolaria;

Am Schädel — On the skull:

 9 Incisura nasoincisiva;
10 Meatus nasi dorsalis;
11 Meatus nasi medius;
12 Foramen infraorbitale;
13 Canalis infraorbitalis;
14 Sinus maxillaris rostralis, rostrale Begrenzung — Sinus maxillaris rostralis, rostral limit;
15 Septum sinuum maxillarium;
16, 17 Sinus maxillaris caudalis:
16 Rostrale Begrenzung — Rostral limit,
17 Kaudoventrale Begrenzung — Caudoventral limit;
18 Hamulus pterygoideus;
19 Apertura frontomaxillaris;
20 Sinus frontalis;
21 Apertura conchofrontalis;
22 Orbita;
23 Fossa sacci lacrimalis;
24 Canalis lacrimalis;
25 Os ethmoidale, Ethmoturbinalia — Os ethmoidale, ethmoturbinates;
26 Ramus mandibulae, rostraler Rand — Ramus mandibulae, rostral border.

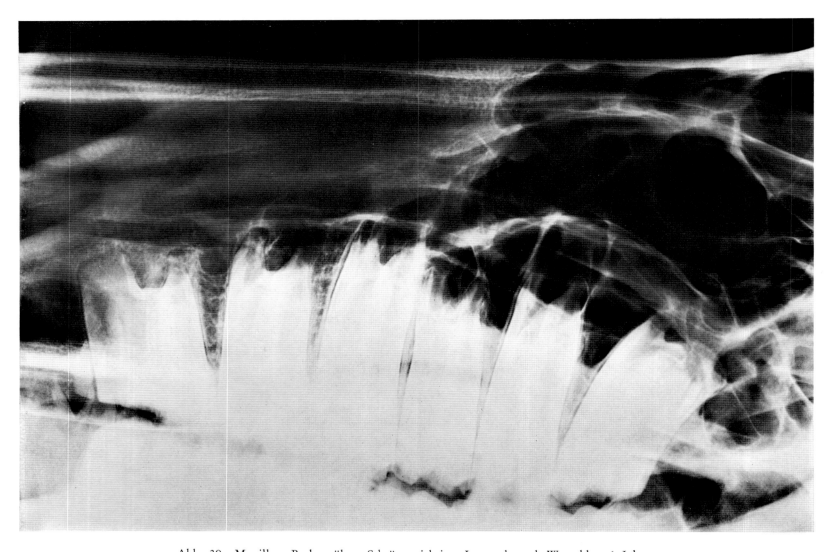

Abb. 39   Maxillare Backenzähne. Schrägprojektion. Latero-lateral. Warmblut, 6 Jahre.
Feinzeichnende Folie — FFA 100 cm — 60 kV — 20 mAs
Verkleinerung von 30 × 40 cm
Lagerung Abb. 30

Fig. 39   Maxillary cheek teeth. Obliquely laterolateral. Light horse, 6 years old.
High definition screens — FFD 100 cm — 60 kV — 20 mAs
Diminution of 30 × 40 cm
Positioning fig. 30

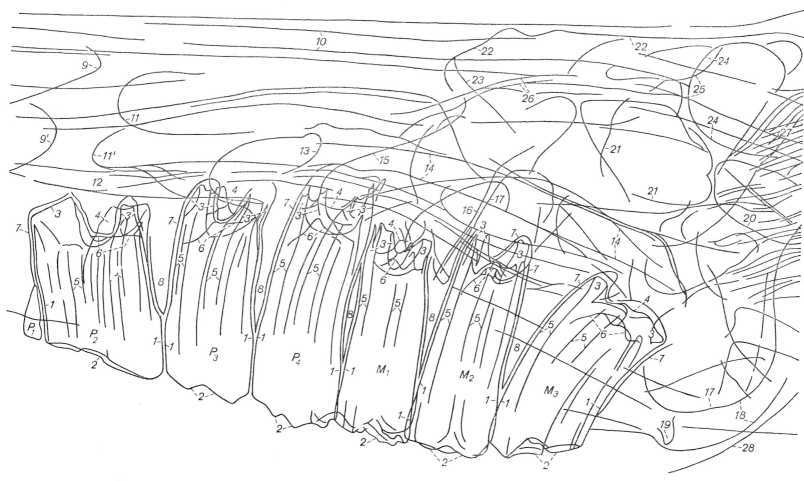

Abb. 40* Röntgenskizze zu Abb. 39   Fig. 40* X-ray sketch to fig. 39

Im Arcus dentalis maxillaris — In the maxillary dental arch:

Dentes permanentes:
P₁ Dens praemolaris I;
P₂ Dens praemolaris II;
P₃ Dens praemolaris III;
P₄ Dens praemolaris IV;
M₁ Dens molaris I;
M₂ Dens molaris II;
M₃ Dens molaris III;

An den maxillaren Backenzähnen — On the maxillary cheek teeth:

1 Corpus dentis;
2 Facies occlusalis et Tubercula coronae dentis;
3 Bukkale Radices dentis — Buccal roots;
4 Palatinale Radix dentis (an M₂ nicht sicher zu identifizieren) — Palatinal root (on M₂ to identify not certainly);
5 Plicae enameli;
6 Infundibula dentis, Grund — Infundibula dentis, base;
7 Alveolus dentalis;
8 Septa interalveolaria;

Am Schädel — On the skull:

9 Incisura nasoincisiva;

10 Meatus nasi dorsalis;
11 Concha nasalis dorsalis;
12 Meatus nasi medius;
13 Foramen infraorbitale;
14 Canalis infraorbitalis;
15 Sinus maxillaris rostralis, rostrale Begrenzung — Sinus maxillaris rostralis, rostral limit;
16 Septum sinuum maxillarium;
17 Sinus maxillaris caudalis, rostrale bzw. kaudoventrale Begrenzung — Sinus maxillaris caudalis, rostral and caudoventral limits respectively;
18 Tuber maxillae;
19 Hamulus pterygoideus;
20 Sinus palatinus;
21 Apertura frontomaxillaris;
22 Sinus frontalis;
23 Sinus conchae dorsalis, rostrale Begrenzung — Sinus conchae dorsalis, rostral limit;
24 Orbita;
25 Fossa sacci lacrimalis;
26 Canalis lacrimalis;
27 Os ethmoidale, Ethmoturbinalia — Os ethmoidale, ethmoturbinates;
28 Ramus mandibulae, rostraler Rand — Ramus mandibulae, rostral border.

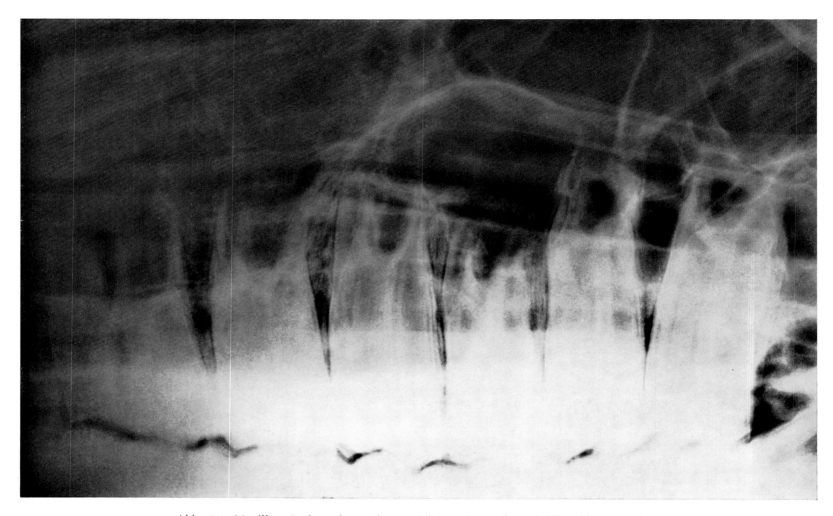

Abb. 41   Maxillare Backenzähne. Schrägprojektion. Latero-lateral. Warmblut, 12 Jahre.
Feinzeichnende Folie — FFA 100 cm — 65 kV — 60 mAs
Originalgröße (Ausschnitt aus 24 × 30 cm)
Lagerung Abb. 30

Fig. 41   Maxillary cheek teeth. Obliquely laterolateral. Light horse, 12 years old.
High definition screens — FFD 100 cm — 65 kV — 60 mAs
Original size (section of 24 × 30 cm)
Positioning fig. 30

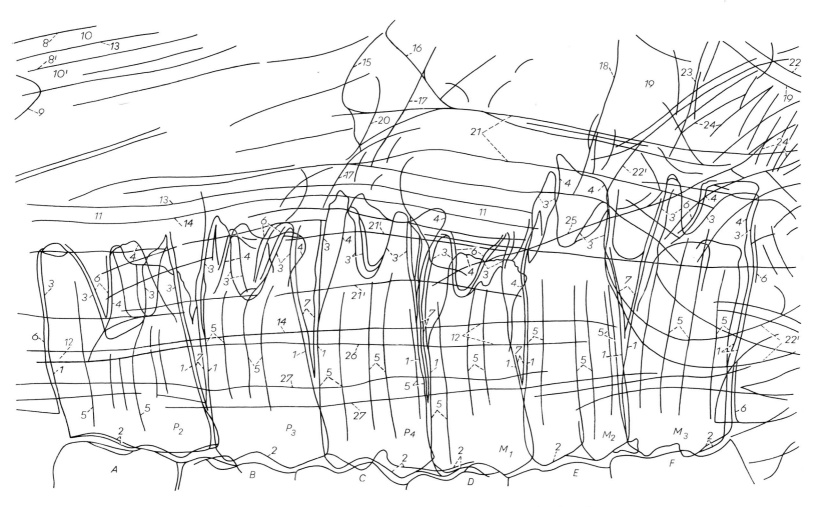

Abb. 42* Röntgenskizze zu Abb. 41   Fig. 42* X-ray sketch to fig. 41

Im Arcus dentalis maxillaris — In the maxillary dental arch:

Dentes permanentes:
P₂ Dens praemolaris II;
P₃ Dens praemolaris III;
P₄ Dens praemolaris IV;
M₁ Dens molaris I;
M₂ Dens molaris II;
M₃ Dens molaris III;

Im Arcus dentalis mandibularis — In the mandibular dental arch:

Dentes permanentes:
A Dens praemolaris II;
B Dens praemolaris III;
C Dens praemolaris IV;
D Dens molaris I;
E Dens molaris II;
F Dens molaris III;

An den maxillaren Backenzähnen — On the maxillary cheek teeth:

1 Corpus dentis;
2 Facies occlusalis;
3 Bukkale Radix dentis — Buccal root;
4 Palatinale Radix dentis — Palatinal root;
5 Verschattungen, die sich aus orthograph getroffenen Abschnitten der Schmelzbecher und aus Plicae enameli ergeben — Shadows formed by orthographically struck parts of the infundibulae and plicae enameli;
6 Alveolus dentalis;
7 Septum interalveolarium;

Am Schädel — On the skull:

8 Os nasale;
9 Incisura nasoincisiva;
10 Meatus nasi dorsalis;
11 Meatus nasi medius;
12 Meatus nasi ventralis;
13 Concha nasalis dorsalis;
14 Concha nasalis ventralis;
15 Sinus conchae dorsalis;
16 Sinus frontalis, rostrale Begrenzung — Sinus frontalis, rostral limit;
17 Sinus maxillaris rostralis;
18 Septum sinuum maxillarium;
19 Sinus maxillaris caudalis;
20 Foramen infraorbitale;
21 Canalis infraorbitalis;
22 Orbita;
23 Os ethmoidale;
24 Ethmoturbinalia;
25 Crista facialis;
26 Palatum durum;
27 Margo alveolaris.

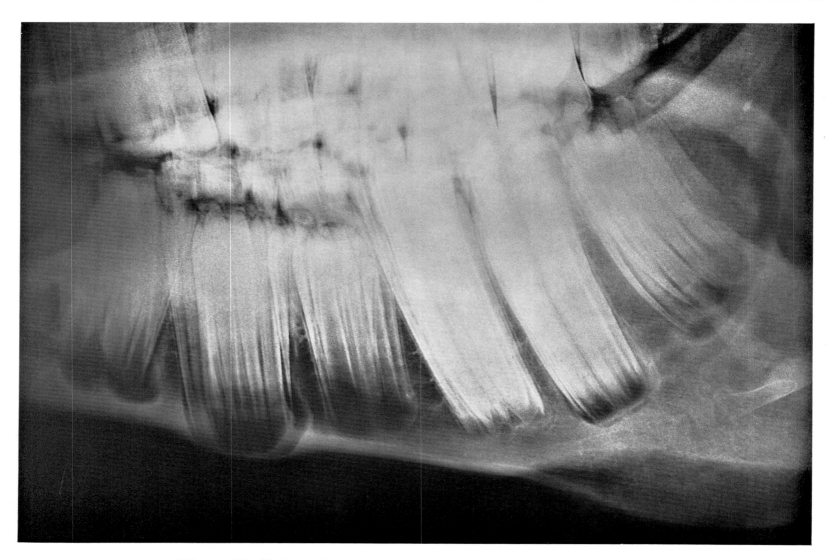

Abb. 43   Mandibulare Backenzähne. Schrägprojektion. Latero-lateral. Traber, 3 Jahre.
Feinzeichnende Folie — FFA 100 cm — 65 kV — 60 mAs
Verkleinerung von 24 × 30 cm
Lagerung Abb. 31

Fig. 43   Mandibular cheek teeth. Obliquely laterolateral. Trotter, 3 years old.
High definition screems — FFD 100 cm — 65 kV — 60 mAs
Diminution of 24 × 30 cm
Positioning fig. 31

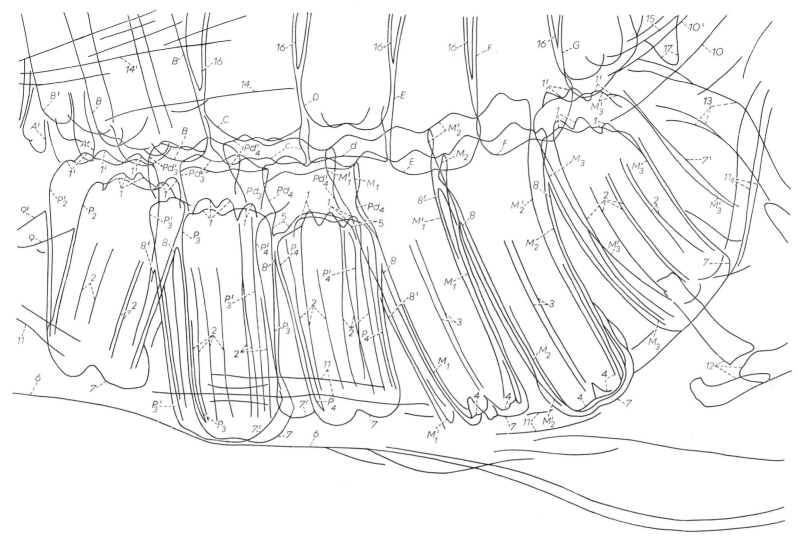

Abb. 44* Röntgenskizze zu Abb. 43 Fig. 44* X-ray sketch to fig. 43

Im Arcus dentalis mandibularis — In the mandibular dental arch:

Dentes permanentes:
P₂ Dens praemolaris II;
P₃ Dens praemolaris III, Anlage — 3rd premolar tooth, primordium;
P₄ Dens praemolaris IV, Anlage — 4th premolar tooth, primordium;
M₁ Dens molaris I;
M₂ Dens molaris II;
M₃ Dens molaris III;

Dentes decidui:
Pd₃ Dens praemolaris deciduus III;
Pd₄ Dens praemolaris deciduus IV;

Im Arcus dentalis maxillaris — In the maxillary dental arch:

Dentes permanentes:
A Dens praemolaris I;
B Dens praemolaris II;
C Dens praemolaris III, Anlage — 3rd premolar tooth, primordium;
D Dens praemolaris IV, Anlage — 4th premolar tooth, primordium;
E Dens molaris I;
F Dens molaris II;
G Dens molaris III;

Dentes decidui:
c Dens praemolaris deciduus III;
d Dens praemolaris deciduus IV;

An den mandibularen Backenzähnen — On the mandibular cheek teeth:
1 Facies occlusalis, Tubercula;
2 Verschattungen, die sich aus den Längsfalten des Schmelzmantels ergeben — Shadows formed by the longitudinal folds of peripheral enamel;
3 Bukkale Längsfurche, orthograph getroffene Abschnitte ihrer seitlichen Begrenzung — Longitudinal buccal groove, orthographically struck parts of its lateral border;
4 Apex radicis dentis permanentis;
5 Radix dentis decidui;

An der Mandibula — On the mandible:
6 Corpus mandibulae;
7 Alveolus dentalis;
8 Septum interalveolarium;
9 Margo interalveolaris;
10 Ramus mandibulae;
11 Canalis mandibulae;

Am Schädel — On the skull:
12 Os hyoideum;
13 Palatum molle;
14 Palatum durum;
15 Tuber maxillae;
16 Septum interalveolarium;
17 Hamulus pterygoideus.

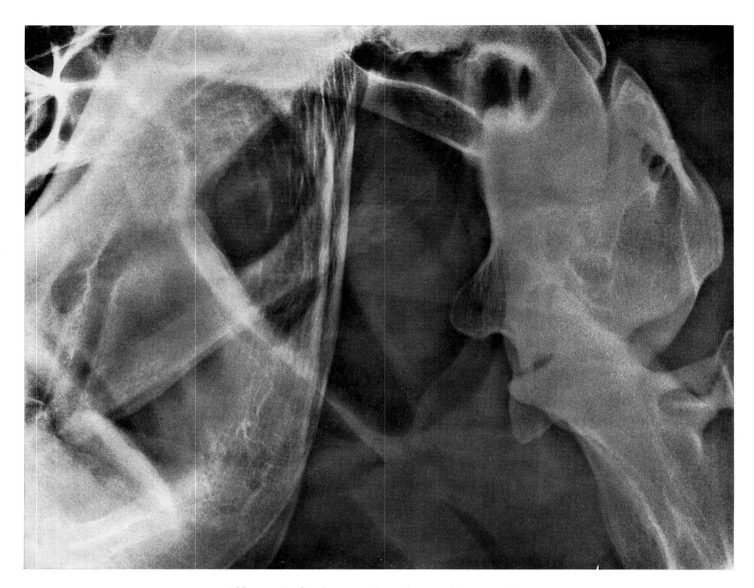

Abb. 45   Luftsack. Latero-lateral. Warmblut, 10 Jahre.
Feinzeichnende Folie — FFA 120 cm — 60 kV — 65 mAs
Verkleinerung von 24 × 30 cm
Lagerung Abb. 32

Fig. 45   Guttural pouch. Laterolateral. Light horse, 10 years old.
High definition screens — FFD 120 cm — 60 kV — 65 mAs
Diminution of 24 × 30 cm
Positioning fig. 32

A   Basis cranii;
B   Ramus mandibulae;
C   Os hyoideum;
D   Atlas;
E   Axis;

a   Articulatio atlantooccipitalis;
b   Articulatio atlantoaxialis;

Am Schädel — On the skull:

1   Sinus maxillaris caudalis;
2   Processus pterygoideus;
3   Os praesphenoidale;
4   Sinus sphenoidalis;
5   Os basisphenoidale;
6   Os occipitale, Pars basilaris;
7   Processus jugularis;
8   Condylus occipitalis;
9   Fossa condylaris ventralis;
10 Canalis nervi hypoglossi;
11 Squama occipitalis;
12 Felsenbeinpyramide — Petrous temporal bone;

13 Fissura petrooccipitalis;
14 Foramen mandibulae;
15 Canalis mandibulae;

Am Os hyoideum — On the hyoid bone:

16 Tympanohyoideum;
17 Stylohyoideum;
18 Basihyoideum;
19 Thyreohyoideum;

Am Atlas — On the atlas:

20 Tuberculum dorsale;
21 Tuberculum ventrale;
22—24   Fovea articularis cranialis:
22 Dorsaler Rand — Dorsal border,
23 Kranialer Rand — Cranial border,
24 Verschattung, die sich aus deren Konkavität ergibt — Shadow formed by its concavity;
25 Foramen vertebrale laterale;
26 Verschattung, die sich aus der Konkavität der Fossa atlantis ergibt — Shadow formed by the concavity of the atlantal fossa;
27 Foramen transversarium;

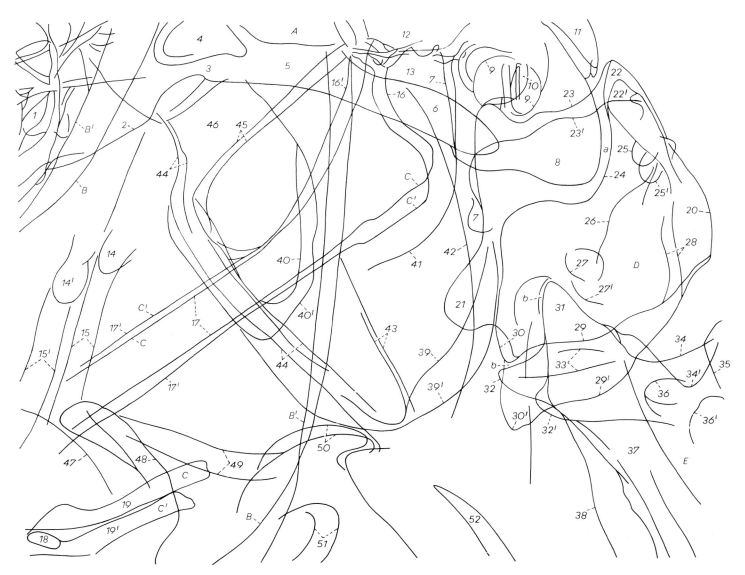

Abb. 46* Röntgenskizze zu Abb. 45 Fig. 46* X-ray sketch to fig. 45

28 Foramen vertebrale, dorsale Begrenzung — Foramen vertebrale, dorsal margin;
29 Fovea articularis caudalis, kaudaler Rand — Fovea articularis caudalis, caudal border;
30 Ala atlantis;

Am Axis — On the axis:

31 Dens;
32 Processus articularis cranialis,
33 Orthograph getroffene Abschnitte — Orthographically struck parts;
34 Arcus vertebrae, kranialer Rand — Arcus vertebrae cranial border;
35 Foramen vertebrale, dorsale Begrenzung — Foramen vertebrale, dorsal margin;
36 Foramen vertebrale laterale;
37 Corpus vertebrae;
38 Crista ventralis;

An Luftsack, Pharynx und Larynx — On the guttural pouch, pharynx and larynx:

39, 40 Diverticulum tubae auditivae:
39 Mediale Bucht — Medial compartment,

40 Laterale Bucht — Lateral compartment;
41 Verschattung, die durch Einfaltung der medialen Bucht von den Nn. glossopharyngeus und hypoglossus entsteht — Shadow formed by invagination of the medial compartment by the glossopharyngeal and hypoglossal nerves;
42 Verschattung, die durch Einfaltung der medialen Bucht von den Nn. vagus und accessorius entsteht — Shadow formed by invagination of the medial compartment by the vagus and accessory nerves;
43 M. longus capitis, ventraler Rand — M. longus capitis, ventral border;
44 Dorsale Pharynxwand — Dorsal wall of pharynx;
45 Tuba auditiva, ventraler Rand des Luftsackabschnitts — Tuba auditiva, ventral border of the diverticular part;
46 Weichteilschatten der Mm. tensor und levator veli palatini — Shadow formed by tensor and levator muscles of the soft palate;
47 Velum palatinum;
48 Epiglottis;
49 Plica aryepiglottica;
50 Cartilago arytaenoidea, Processus corniculatus;
51 Ventriculus laryngis lateralis;
52 Oesophagus, lufthaltiger Abschnitt — Esophagus, air-containing part.

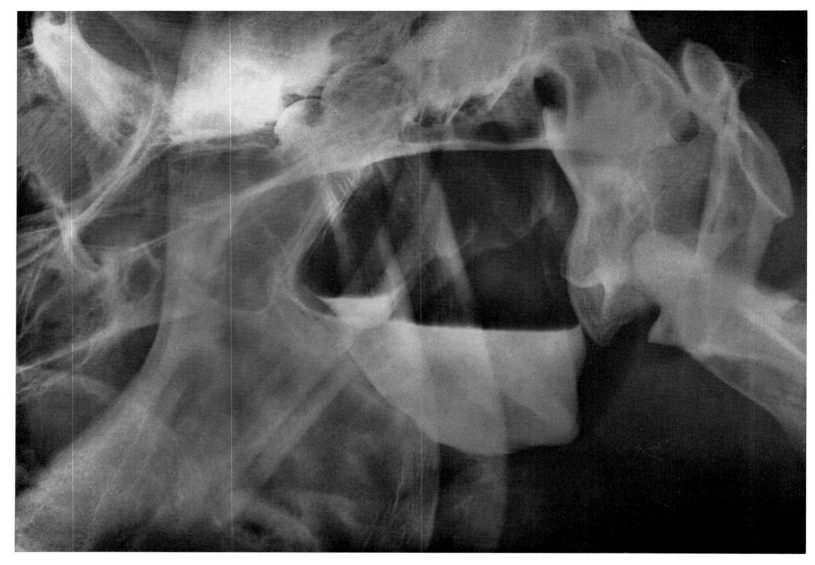

Abb. 47 Luftsack, einseitige Kontrastfüllung, rechts (Kaliumjodid, 10%ig). Latero-lateral. Kleinpferd, 23 Jahre.
Feinzeichnende Folie — FFA 120 cm — 65 kV — 70 mAs
Originalgröße (Ausschnitt aus 24 × 30 cm)
Lagerung Abb. 32

Fig. 47 Guttural pouch, contrast medium, unilateral, right side (10 % potassium iodide). Laterolateral. Pony, 23 years old.
High definition screens — FFD 120 cm — 65 kV — 70 mAs
Original size (section of 24 × 30 cm)
Positioning fig. 32

A   Schädel — Skull;
B   Ramus mandibulae;
C   Os hyoideum;
D   Atlas;
E   Axis;
M_3 Mandibularer Dens molaris III — 3rd mandibular molar tooth;

a   Articulatio temporomandibularis;
b   Articulatio atlantooccipitalis;
c   Articulatio atlantoaxialis;

Am Schädel — On the skull:

1   Os frontale, Processus zygomaticus;
2   Knochenleiste an der medialen Seite von 1 — Bone ridge on the medial wall of 1;
3   Crista facialis;
4   Os temporale, Processus zygomaticus;
5   Labyrinthus ethmoidalis;
6   Lamina cribrosa;
7   Sinus maxillaris;
8   Tuber maxillae;
9   Os pterygoideum, zugleich seitliche Begrenzung der Choane — Os pterygoideum forming the lateral border of the choana;
10   Hamulus pterygoideus;
11   Fossa pterygopalatina;
12   Os palatinum, zugleich kaudale Begrenzung der Choane — Os palatinum forming the caudal border of the choana;

13   Processus pterygoideus;
14   Sinus palatinus;
15   Sinus sphenoidalis;
16   Canalis opticus et Foramen opticum;
17   Os basisphenoidale;
18   Os occipitale, Pars basilaris;
19   Condylus occipitalis;
20   Processus jugularis;
21   Fossa condylaris ventralis;
22   Canalis nervi hypoglossi;
23   Squama occipitalis;
24   Felsenbeinpyramide — Petrous temporal bone;
25   Fissura petrooccipitalis;
26   Foramen lacerum, rostraler Rand — Foramen lacerum, rostral margin;
27   Processus retroarticularis;
28   Fossa mandibularis;
29   Verschattung, die sich aus dem Tuberculum articulare ergibt — Shadow formed by the articular tuberosity;
30   Processus condylaris;
31   Processus coronoideus;
32   Canalis mandibulae, rostrale Begrenzung — Canalis mandibulae, rostral border;

Am Os hyoideum — On the hyoid bone:

33   Stylohyoideum;
34   Tympanohyoideum;

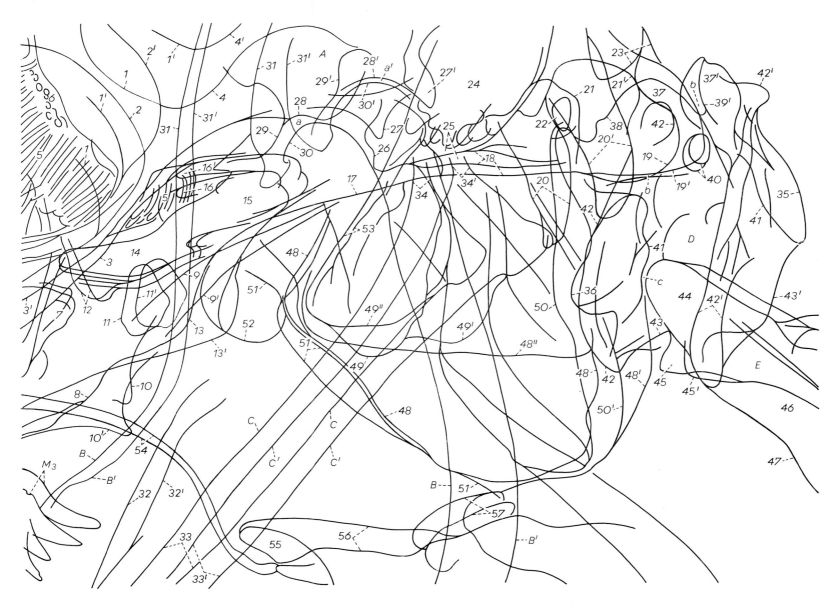

Abb. 48* Röntgenskizze zu Abb. 47   Fig. 48* X-ray sketch to fig. 47

Am Atlas — On the atlas:

35   Tuberculum dorsale;
36   Tuberculum ventrale;
37—39   Fovea articularis cranialis:
37   Dorsaler Rand — Dorsal border,
38   Kranialer Rand — Cranial border,
39   Verschattung, die sich aus deren Konkavität ergibt — Shadow formed by its concavity;
40   Foramen vertebrale laterale;
41   Foramen vertebrale, dorsale bzw. ventrale Begrenzung — Foramen vertebrale, dorsal and ventral margins respectively;
42   Ala atlantis;
43   Fovea articularis caudalis, kaudaler Rand — Fovea articularis caudalis, caudal border;

Am Axis — On the axis:

44   Dens;
45   Processus articularis cranialis;
46   Corpus vertebrae;
47   Crista ventralis;

An Luftsack, Pharynx und Larynx — On the guttural pouch, pharynx and larynx:

48, 49   Diverticulum tubae auditivae:
48   Mediale Bucht — Medial compartment,
49   Laterale Bucht — Lateral compartment;
48″, 49″   Kontrastmittelspiegel — Contrast medium level;
50   Verschattung, die durch Einfaltung der medialen Bucht von den Nn. vagus und accessorius entsteht — Shadow formed by invagination of the medial compartment by the vagus and accessory nerves;
51   Dorsale Pharynxwand — Dorsal wall of the pharynx;
52   Kontrastmittelschatten, am Rand des Ostium pharyngeum tubae auditivae — Shadow formed by the contrast medium at the margin of the pharyngeal opening of the auditory tube;
53   Kontrastmittelschatten am ventralen Rand des Luftsackabschnitts der Tuba auditiva — Shadow of the contrast medium at the ventral margin of the diverticular part of the auditory tube;
54   Velum palatinum;
55   Epiglottis;
56   Plica aryepiglottica;
57   Cartilago arytaenoidea, Processus corniculatus.

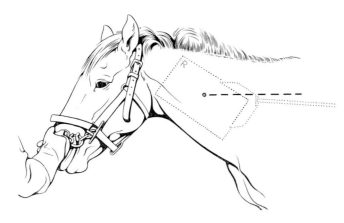

Abb. 49   Lagerung zur Aufnahme der Halswirbelsäule. Latero-lateral.
Die Untersuchung des 1. bis 5. Halswirbels ist am stehenden Pferd möglich. Schwierigkeiten ergeben sich bei der Einstellung des Zentralstrahls
und der Ausblendung. Daraus resultiert, daß in dieser Position eine
Bucky-Blende nur in Ausnahmefällen angewendet werden kann. Wegen
der erforderlichen hohen Spannung mindert die Streustrahlung die
Bildqualität.
Der Zentralstrahl sollte den Hals in Höhe des 2. bzw. 4. Halswirbels
treffen und im rechten Winkel auf die Kassette einfallen.

Fig. 49   Positioning of cervical vertebral column. Laterolateral.
Radiography of the 1st to the 5th cervical vertebrae is possible in a
standing horse. Difficulties are experienced in directing the central beam
and setting the shutter. Consequently a Bucky diaphragm can be employed only in exceptional cases. Because of the high tension, necessary,
scattered radiation diminishes the quality of the radiograph.
The central beam should strike the neck on a level of the 2nd or 4th
vertebra respectively, and fall at right angles to the cassette.

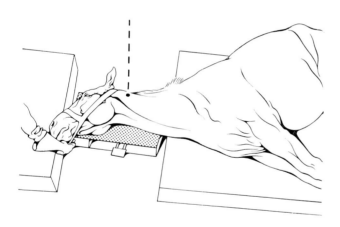

Abb. 50   Lagerung zur Aufnahme der Halswirbelsäule
(1. bis 3. Halswirbel). Latero-lateral.
Bei der Lagerung ist zu beachten, daß sich die Oberfläche des Kastens
mit der eingebauten Bucky-Blende in gleicher Höhe zur Oberfläche der
Matte, auf der das Pferd liegt, befindet. Kopf und Hals sind leicht gestreckt zu lagern. Es ist ein großes Filmformat zu verwenden und sorgfältig auszublenden.
Wenn keine Bucky-Blende verfügbar ist, kann eine Kassette mit stehendem Raster zur Verminderung der Streustrahlung verwendet werden.
Der Zentralstrahl sollte den Hals etwa handbreit kaudal des Atlasflügels
treffen und im rechten Winkel auf die Kassette einfallen.

Fig. 50   Positioning of cervical vertebral column
(1st to 3rd cervical vertebrae). Laterolateral.
In this positioning, it is necessary to ensure that the top of the box with
the built-in Bucky diaphragm remains at the same level as the mat on
which the horse is placed. The head and neck should be stretched slightly.
A film of a large size should be used and the setting of the shutter must
be exact.
To reduce scattered radiation, a cassette with a stationary grid may be
used instead of a Bucky diaphragm.
The central beam should strike the neck approximately a hands' breadth
caudal to the wing of the atlas and fall at right angles to the cassette.

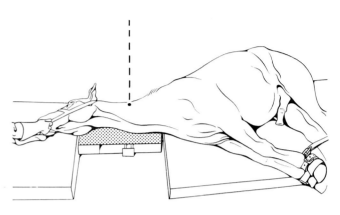

Abb. 51   Lagerung zur Aufnahme der Halswirbelsäule
(3. bis 6. Halswirbel). Latero-lateral.
Schwierigkeiten ergeben sich bei der korrekten Lagerung des Halses auf
der Bucky-Blende. Da Kopf und Brust breiter als der zu untersuchende
Halsbereich sind, hängt die Halswirbelsäule gering konkav durch. Daraus können in krassen Fällen Verzeichnungen und damit Schwierigkeiten bei der Interpretation der Aufnahme resultieren.
Bei der Lagerung des Pferdes ist darauf zu achten, daß die Schultergliedmaßen ausreichend nach kaudal gezogen, Kopf und Hals gestreckt fixiert
werden und sich die Oberfläche des Blendenkastens in gleicher Höhe zu
der Matte befindet.
Wenn keine Bucky-Blende verfügbar ist, kann zur Verminderung der
Streustrahlung eine Kassette mit stehendem Raster verwendet werden.
Es ist zweckmäßig, ein großes Filmformat zu wählen.
Der Zentralstrahl sollte den Hals 3—4fingerbreit dorsal der Trachea in
Höhe des 4. Halswirbels treffen und im rechten Winkel auf die Kas-
sette einfallen.

Fig. 51   Positioning of cervical vertebral column
(3rd to 6th cervical vertebrae). Laterolateral.
Difficulties arise in the proper positioning of the neck on the Bucky
diaphragm. Because the thickness of the head and the breast is greater
than the thickness of the neck, the cervical spine remains in a slightly
concave position. In marked cases, this could result in distortions and
difficulties in interpretation.
In positioning the horse, care must be exercised to stretch the front limbs
sufficiently caudally, to extend and stabilize the head and neck, and to
keep the top of the Bucky diaphragm on the same level as the mat.
To reduce scattered radiation, a cassette with stationary grid may be used
instead of a Bucky diaphragm.
A film of large size should be used.
The central beam should strike the neck at a width of 3—4 fingers dorsally to the trachea on a level of the 4th cervical vertebra and fall at
right angles to the cassette.

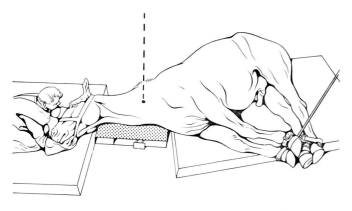

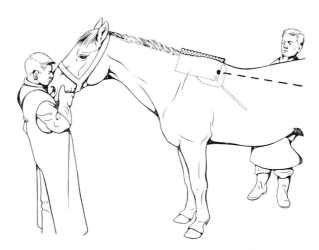

Abb. 52 Lagerung zur Aufnahme der Halswirbelsäule
(4. Halswirbel bis 1. Brustwirbel). Latero-lateral.

Das Pferd ist mit weit nach hinten gezogenen Schultergliedmaßen so zu lagern, daß der Widerrist und das Schultergelenk an der Mattenkante liegen. Kopf und Hals sind gestreckt zu fixieren. Die Oberfläche des Blendenkastens sollte zweifingerbreit über, zumindest aber in gleicher Höhe der Mattenoberfläche liegen, um einer Wölbung der Halswirbelsäule und den daraus resultierenden Schwierigkeiten bei der Interpretation vorzubeugen.
Wenn keine Bucky-Blende verfügbar ist, kann zur Verminderung der Streustrahlung eine Kassette mit stehendem Raster verwendet werden. Der Zentralstrahl sollte den Hals in Höhe des 5. Halswirbels (etwa eine Handlänge kranial der 1. Rippe und handbreit dorsal der Trachea) treffen und im rechten Winkel auf die Kassette einfallen.

Fig. 52 Positioning of cervical vertebral column
(4th cervical to 1st thoracic vertebrae). Laterolateral.

The horse, with front limbs pulled far caudally, must be placed in such a manner that the withers and the shoulder joint rest on the edge of the mat. The head and neck must be fixed in an extended position. The top of the Bucky box should be the width of 2 fingers above the top of the mat, or at least at the same level of the latter to avoid arching of the cervical spine and difficulties in interpretation that might result from it.
In order to reduce scattered radiation, a cassette with a stationary grid may be used instead of a Bucky diaphragm.
The central beam should strike the neck on a level of the 5th cervical vertebra approximately a hand's length cranial to the 1st rib and the width of a hand dorsal to the trachea, and fall at right angles to the cassette.

Abb. 53 Lagerung zur Aufnahme der Widerristdornfortsätze.
Latero-lateral.

Bei dieser Lagerung sind die freien Enden der Dornfortsätze darzustellen. Wegen der starken Rückenmuskulatur (Strahlenabsorption, Streustrahlung) und wegen des relativ großen Objekt-Film-Abstands sind brauchbare Aufnahmen der Dornfortsatzbasis nur am liegenden Tier bei Verwendung einer Bucky-Blende bzw. einer Kassette mit stehendem Raster zu erhalten.
Die Kassette ist parallel zur Medianebene zu lagern.
Der Zentralstrahl sollte den Widerrist etwa handbreit ventral der Rückenkontur in Höhe des zu untersuchenden Dornfortsatzes treffen und im rechten Winkel auf die Kassette einfallen.

Fig. 53 Positioning of spinous processes of the withers.
Laterolateral.

The free ends of the spinous processes can be depicted in this position. Because of the well developed spinal musculature (absorption of the rays, scattered radiation) and a relatively great object-to-film distance, radiographs of the base of the spinous process can only be obtained in the recumbent animal, using a Bucky diaphragm or a cassette with a stationary grid.
The central beam should strike the withers approximately a handwidth ventrally to the backline on a level of the spinous process to be examined and fall at right angles to the cassette.

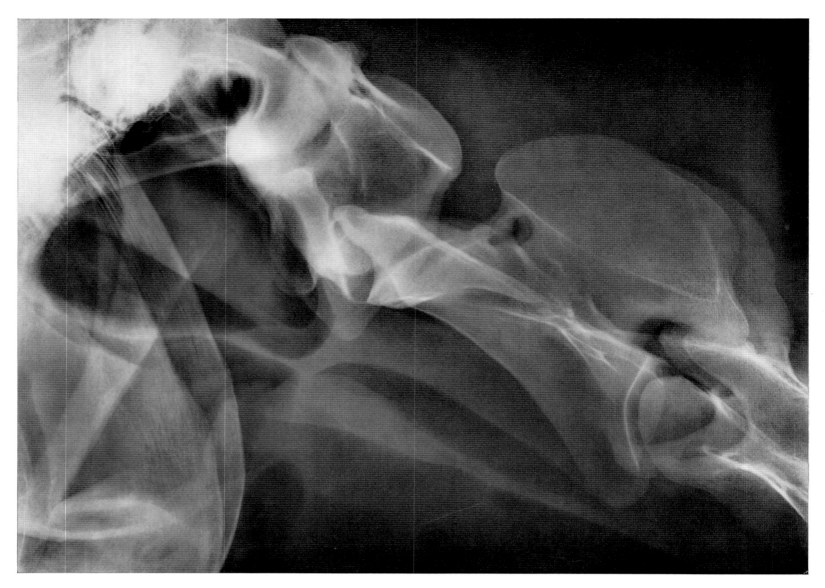

Abb. 54   Halswirbelsäule (1. bis 3. Halswirbel). Latero-lateral. Warmblut, 13 Jahre.
Bucky-Blende — Feinzeichnende Folie — FFA 100 cm — 95 kV — 50 mAs
Verkleinerung von 30 × 40 cm
Lagerung Abb. 50

Fig. 54   Cervical vertebral column (1st to 3rd cervical vertebrae). Laterolateral. Light horse, 13 years old.
Bucky diaphragm — High definition screens — FFD 100 cm — 95 kV — 50 mAs
Diminution of 30 × 40 cm
Positioning fig. 50

A   Cranium;
B   Mandibula;
C   Os hyoideum;
D   Atlas;
E   Axis;
F   3. Vertebra cervicalis;
G   Larynx;
H   Trachea;

a   Articulatio temporomandibularis;
b   Articulatio atlantooccipitalis;
c   Articulatio atlantoaxialis;

Am Schädel — On the skull:

1   Os occipitale, Partes laterales, zugleich dorsale Begrenzung des Foramen magnum — Os occipitale, partes laterales, forming the dorsal margin of the foramen magnum;
2   Condylus occipitalis;
3   Processus jugularis;
4   Os occipitale, Pars basilaris, zugleich ventrale Begrenzung des Foramen magnum — Os occipitale, pars basilaris, forming the ventral margin of the foramen magnum;
5   Canalis nervi hypoglossi, seine Begrenzung abschnittsweise dargestellt — Canalis nervi hypoglossi, its border shown partly;
6   Felsenbeinpyramide — Petrous temporal bone;

7   Processus styloideus;
8   Fissura petrooccipitalis;
9   Processus condylaris;
10   Canalis mandibulae;

Am Os hyoideum — On the hyoid bone:

11   Tympanohyoideum;
12   Stylohyoideum;
13   Thyreohyoideum;

Am Atlas — On the atlas:

14   Arcus dorsalis et Tuberculum dorsale;
15   Arcus ventralis et Tuberculum ventrale (15″);
16   Foramen vertebrale, dorsale bzw. ventrale Begrenzung — Foramen vertebrale, dorsal and ventral margins respectively;
17, 18   Fovea articularis cranialis:
17   Kranialer Rand — Cranial border,
18   Kaudaler Rand — Caudal border;
19   Ala atlantis;
20   Verschattung, die sich aus der Konkavität der Fossa atlantis ergibt — Shadow formed by the concavity of the atlantal fossa;
21   Verschattungen, die sich aus der Konkavität des Foramen alare ergeben und zugleich seine kraniale und kaudale Begrenzung sind — Shadows formed by the concavity of the alar foramen and also forming its cranial and caudal margins;

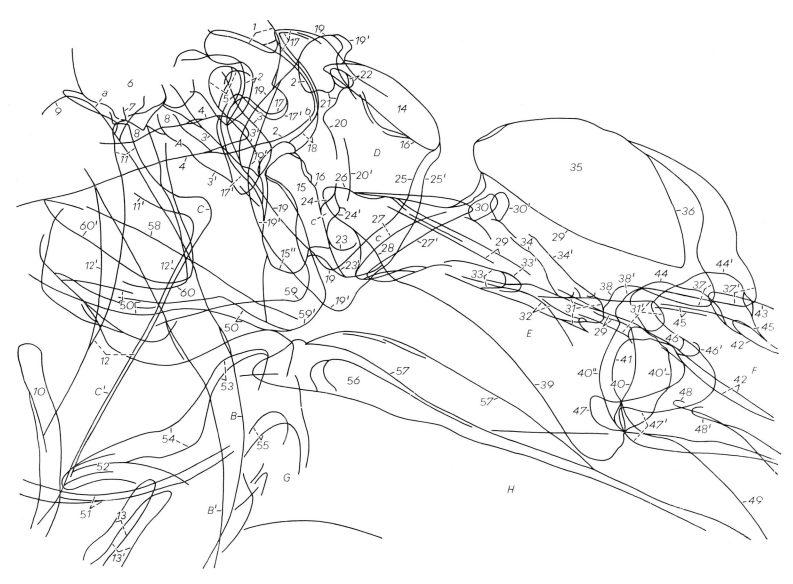

Abb. 55* Röntgenskizze zu Abb. 54   Fig. 55* X-ray sketch to fig. 54

22 Foramen vertebrale laterale;
23 Verschattung, die sich aus der Basis der Fovea articularis cranialis sowie der Ala atlantis ergibt, die bei 24 das Foramen transversum kaudal begrenzt — Shadow formed by the base of the cranial articular fovea and the wing of the atlas, bordering the transverse foramen caudally at 24;
25 Fovea articularis caudalis, kaudaler Rand — Fovea articularis caudalis, caudal border;

Am Axis — On the axis:

26 Dens;
27 Processus articularis cranialis;
28 Verschattung, die sich aus der Konkavität der Rinne zwischen den Processus articulares craniales ergibt — Shadow formed by the groove between the cranial articular processes;
29 Foramen vertebrale, ventrale bzw. dorsale Begrenzung — Foramen vertebrale, ventral and dorsal margins respectively;
30 Foramen vertebrale laterale;
31 Processus transversus;
32 Verschattungen, die sich aus der Basis des Processus transversus ergeben — Shadows formed by the base of the transverse process;
33 Foramen transversarium;
34 Kompaktaverstärkung am Arcus vertebrae — Increased compacta of the vertebral arch;
35 Processus spinosus;
36 Verschattung, die sich aus der Konkavität der Rinne zwischen den beiden Processus articulares caudales ergibt — Shadow formed by the concavity of the groove between the caudal articular processes;
37 Processus articularis caudalis;
38 Incisura vertebralis caudalis;
39 Crista ventralis;
40 Extremitas caudalis,
40″ Verschattung, die sich aus ihrer Konkavität ergibt — Shadow formed by its concavity;

Am 3. Halswirbel — On the 3rd cervical vertebra:

41 Extremitas cranialis;
42 Foramen vertebrale, ventrale bzw. dorsale Begrenzung — Foramen vertebrale, ventral and dorsal margins respectively;
43 Processus spinosus;
44 Processus articularis cranialis;
45 Verschattung, die sich aus der Kompaktaverstärkung am Processus articularis cranialis ergibt und in die Kompaktaverstärkung aus der Wölbung des Arcus vertebrae beiderseits vom Processus spinosus übergeht — Shadow formed by the increased compacta of the cranial articular process and blending with the increased compacta formed by the curvature of the vertebral arch on either side of the spinous process;
46 Incisura vertebralis cranialis;
47 Processus transversus, Tuberculum ventrale;
48 Verschattung, die sich aus der Basis des Processus transversus ergibt — Shadow formed by the base of the transverse process;
49 Crista ventralis;

An Pharynx und Larynx — On the pharynx and larynx:

50 Dorsale Pharynxwand — Dorsal wall of the pharynx;
51 Arcus palatopharyngeus;
52 Epiglottis;
53 Cartilago arytaenoidea, Processus corniculatus;
54 Plica aryepiglottica;
55 Ventriculus laryngis lateralis;
56 Cartilago cricoidea, Lamina;
57 Oesophagus, lufthaltiger Abschnitt — Esophagus, air-containing part;
58 M. longus capitis, ventraler Rand — M. longus capitis, ventral border;
59, 60 Diverticulum tubae auditivae:
59 Laterale Bucht — Lateral compartment,
60 Mediale Bucht — Medial compartment.

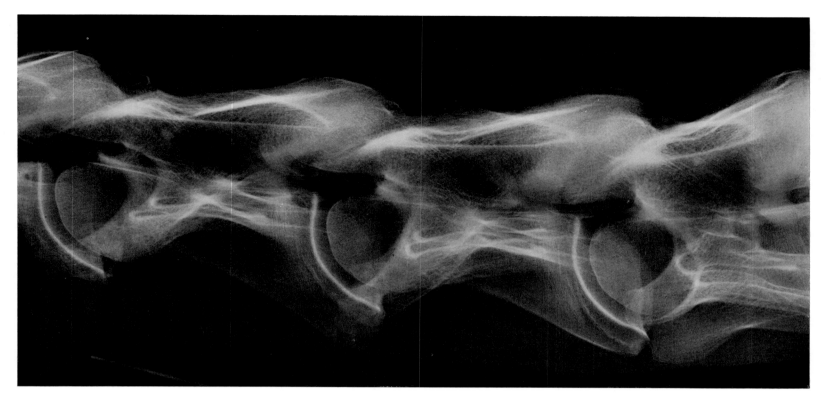

Abb. 56   Halswirbelsäule (3. bis 6. Halswirbel). Latero-lateral. Warmblut, 3 Jahre.
Bucky-Blende — Feinzeichnende Folie — FFA 100 cm — 85 kV — 90 mAs
Verkleinerung von 30 × 40 cm
Lagerung Abb. 51

Fig. 56   Cervical vertebral column (3rd to 6th cervical vertebrae). Laterolateral. Light horse, 3 years old.
Bucky diaphragm — High definition screens — FFD 100 cm — 85 kV — 90 mAs
Diminution of 30 × 40 cm
Positioning fig. 51

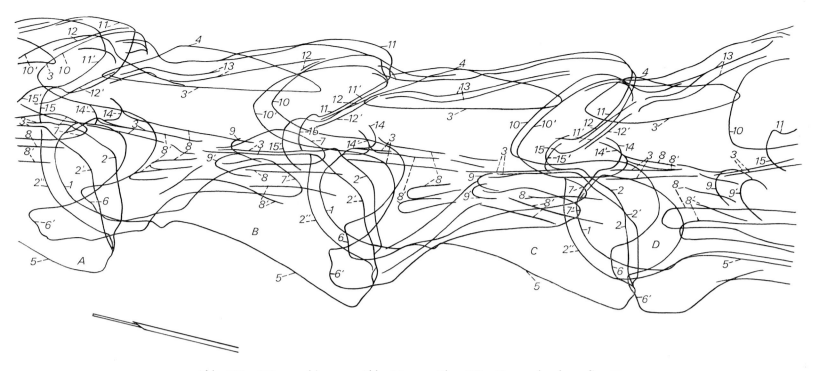

Abb. 57*   Röntgenskizze zu Abb. 56   Fig. 57*   X-ray sketch to fig. 56

A   3. Vertebra cervicalis;
B   4. Vertebra cervicalis;
C   5. Vertebra cervicalis;
D   6. Vertebra cervicalis;

1   Extremitas cranialis;
2   Extremitas caudalis,
2″   Verschattung, die sich aus ihrer Konkavität ergibt — Shadow formed by its concavity;
3   Foramen vertebrale, ventrale bzw. dorsale Begrenzung — Foramen vertebrale, ventral and dorsal margins respectively;
4   Processus spinosus;
5   Crista ventralis;
6, 7 Processus transversus:
6   Tuberculum ventrale,
7   Tuberculum dorsale;
8   Verschattungen, die sich aus der Basis des Processus transversus ergeben, zugleich ventrale bzw. dorsale Begrenzung des Foramen

transversarium — Shadows formed by the base of the transverse process, also forming the ventral and dorsal margins of the transverse foramen respectively;
9   Foramen transversarium, kaudolateraler Rand — Foramen transversarium, caudolateral margin;
10   Processus articularis cranialis;
11   Processus articularis caudalis;
12   Verschattungen, die sich aus der Konkavität der Gelenkflächen ergeben — Shadows formed by the concavity of the articular surfaces;
13   Verschattungen, die sich aus der Wölbung des Arcus vertebrae beiderseits vom Processus spinosus ergeben — Shadows formed by the curvature of the vertebral arch on either side of the spinous process;
14, 15 Incisurae vertebrales cranialis et caudalis, die das Foramen intervertebrale begrenzen — Incisurae vertebrales cranialis et caudalis bordering the intervertebral foramen.

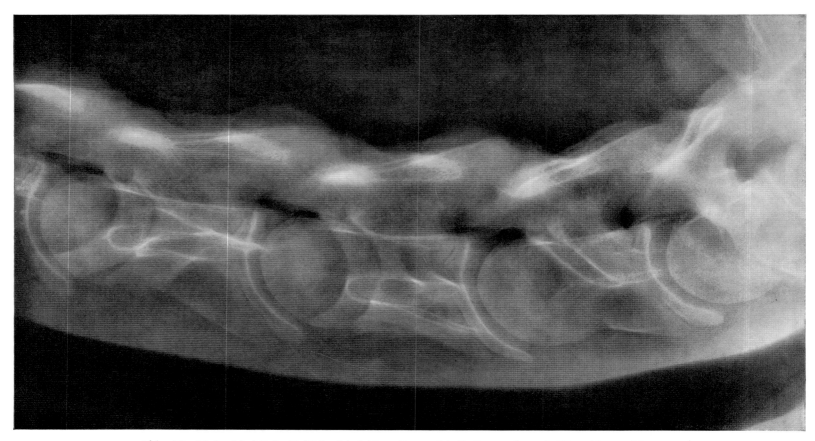

Abb. 58   Halswirbelsäule (4. Halswirbel bis 1. Brustwirbel). Latero-lateral. Warmblut, 8 Monate.
Bucky-Blende — Feinzeichnende Folie — FFA 100 cm — 75 kV — 150 mAs
Verkleinerung von 30 × 40 cm
Lagerung Abb. 52

Fig. 58   Cervical vertebral column (4th cervical to 1st thoracic vertebrae). Laterolateral. Light horse, 8 months old.
Bucky diaphragm — High definition screens — FFD 100 cm — 75 kV — 150 mAs
Diminution of 30 × 40 cm
Positioning fig. 52

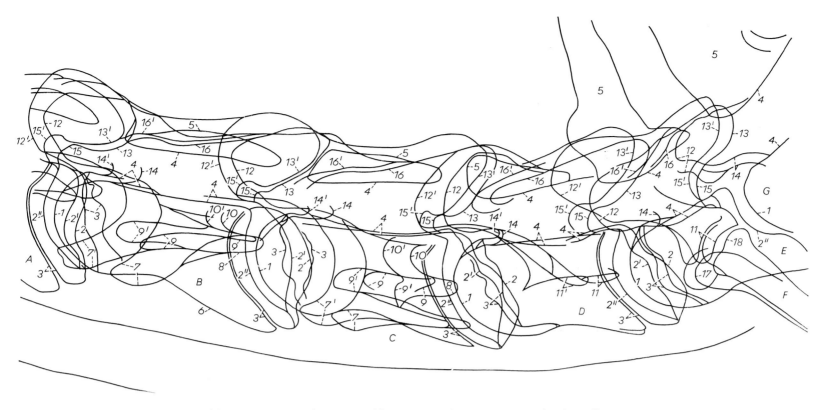

Abb. 59* Röntgenskizze zu Abb. 58   Fig. 59* X-ray sketch to fig. 58

A   4. Vertebra cervicalis;
B   5. Vertebra cervicalis;
C   6. Vertebra cervicalis;
D   7. Vertebra cervicalis;
E   1. Vertebra thoracica;
F   1. Os costale;
G   2. Vertebra thoracica;

1   Extremitas cranialis;
2   Extremitas caudalis;
2″ Verschattung, die sich aus ihrer Konkavität ergibt — Shadow formed by its concavity;
3   Epiphysenfuge — Epiphyseal cartilage;
4   Foramen vertebrale, ventrale bzw. dorsale Begrenzung — Foramen vertebrale, ventral and dorsal margins respectively;
5   Processus spinosus;
6   Crista ventralis;
7, 8   Processus transversus:
7   Tuberculum ventrale,
8   Tuberculum dorsale;

9   Verschattung, die sich aus der Basis des Processus transversus ergibt, die dorsale Verschattung ist zugleich der Boden des Foramen transversarium — Shadow formed by the base of the transverse process, the dorsal shadow also forming the base of the transverse foramen;
10   Foramen transversarium, kaudaler Rand — Foramen transversarium, caudal margin;
11   Verschattung, die sich aus der Basis des Processus transversus am 7. Hals- und 1. Brustwirbel ergibt — Shadow formed by the base of the transverse process of the 7th cervical and 1st thoracic vertebrae;
12   Processus articularis cranialis;
13   Processus articularis caudalis;
14, 15   Incisurae vertebrales cranialis et caudalis, die das Foramen intervertebrale begrenzen — Incisurae vertebrales cranialis et caudalis bordering the intervertebral foramen;
16   Verschattungen, die sich aus der Wölbung des Arcus vertebrae beiderseits vom Processus spinosus ergeben — Shadows formed by the curvature of the vertebral arch on either side of the spinous process;
17   Caput costae;
18   Tuberculum costae.

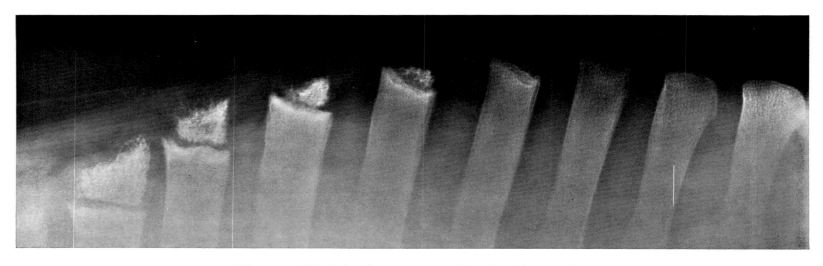

Abb. 60   Widerristdornfortsätze. Latero-lateral. Traber, 6 Jahre.
Feinzeichnende Folie — FFA 100 cm — 55 kV — 35 mAs
Verkleinerung von 15 × 40 cm
Lagerung Abb. 53

Fig. 60   Spinous processes of the withers. Laterolateral. Trotter, 6 years old.
High definition screens — FFD 100 cm — 55 kV — 35 mAs
Diminution of 15 × 40 cm
Positioning fig. 53

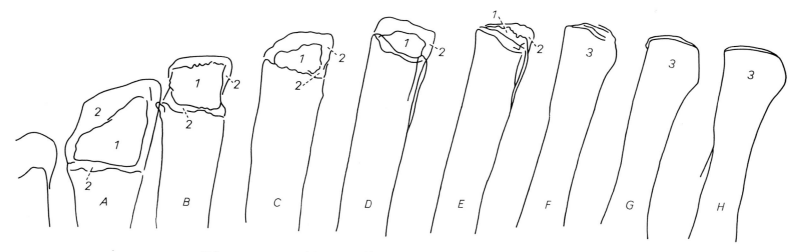

Abb. 61   Röntgenskizze zu Abb. 60   Fig. 61   X-ray sketch to fig. 60

A   3. Vertebra thoracica, Processus spinosus;
B   4. Vertebra thoracica, Processus spinosus;
C   5. Vertebra thoracica, Processus spinosus;
D   6. Vertebra thoracica, Processus spinosus;
E   7. Vertebra thoracica, Processus spinosus;
F   8. Vertebra thoracica, Processus spinosus;
G   9. Vertebra thoracica, Processus spinosus;
H   10. Vertebra thoracica, Processus spinosus;

1—3 Tuberositas spinosa:
1   Knochenkern — Center of ossification,
2   Knorpelschatten — Shadow formed by the cartilage,
3   Verknöchert — Ossified.

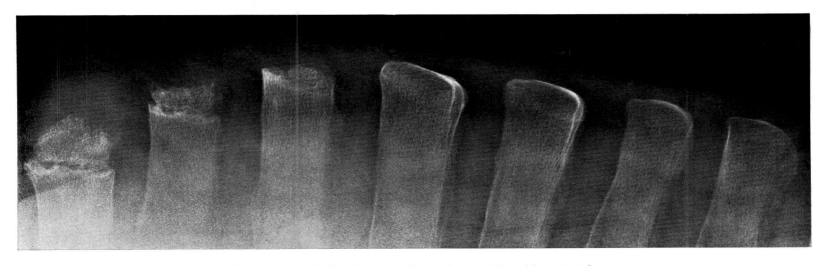

Abb. 62   Widerristdornfortsätze. Latero-lateral. Warmblut, 12 Jahre.
Feinzeichnende Folie — FFA 120 cm — 58 kV — 35 mAs
Verkleinerung von 15 × 40 cm
Lagerung Abb. 53

Fig. 62   Spinous processes of the withers. Laterolateral. Light horse, 12 years old.
High definition screens — FFD 120 cm — 58 kV — 35 mAs
Diminution of 15 × 40 cm
Positioning fig. 53

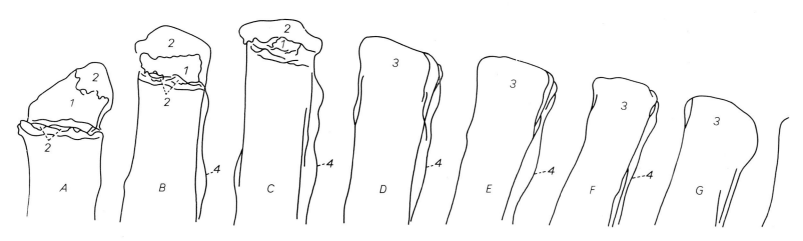

Abb. 63   Röntgenskizze zu Abb. 62   Fig. 63   X-ray sketch to fig. 62

A	3. Vertebra thoracica, Processus spinosus;
B	4. Vertebra thoracica, Processus spinosus;
C	5. Vertebra thoracica, Processus spinosus;
D	6. Vertebra thoracica, Processus spinosus;
E	7. Vertebra thoracica, Processus spinosus;
F	8. Vertebra thoracica, Processus spinosus;
G	9. Vertebra thoracica, Processus spinosus;

1—4 Tuberositas spinosa:
1   Knochenkern — Center of ossification,
2   Knorpelschatten — Shadow formed by the cartilage,
3   Verknöchert — Ossified,
4   Knochenleiste am kaudalen Rand — Bone ridge on the caudal border.

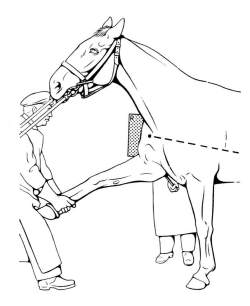

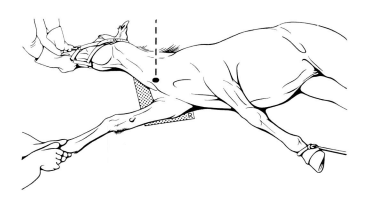

Abb. 64 Lagerung zur Aufnahme des Schultergelenks, stehend.
Medio-lateral.

Die Anfertigung einer Aufnahme am stehenden Pferd ist nur möglich, wenn die dabei verursachten Schmerzen unbedeutend bleiben bzw. die Schmerzen und die Abwehr gegen die unnatürliche Gliedmaßenfixierung durch eine Sedierung ausgeschaltet werden können. Wesentlich ist, daß die Gliedmaße nicht nur hochgehoben, sondern auch nach vorn gezogen und der Kopf des Pferdes möglichst hoch gehalten werden. Zur Verringerung der Streustrahlung ist eine Kassette mit stehendem Raster zu verwenden.
Der Zentralstrahl sollte die Mitte des Gelenks in Höhe des Tuberculum majus treffen und im rechten Winkel auf die Kassette einfallen.

Fig. 64 Positioning of shoulder joint, standing. Mediolateral.

Radiography of a horse in the standing position is possible only when the resulting pain remains insignificant or when the pain and the resistance against an unnatural fixation of the extremity can be eliminated with the help of sedation. It is essential that the limb not only be held high, but also be pulled forward and the head be held as high as possible.
In order to reduce scattered radiation a cassette with a stationary grid should be used.
The central beam should strike the center of the joint on a level of the tuberculum majus and fall at right angles to the cassette.

Abb. 65 Lagerung zur Aufnahme des Schultergelenks, liegend.
Medio-lateral.

Die zu untersuchende (untenliegende) Gliedmaße ist weit nach vorn, die obenliegende weit nach hinten zu fixieren. Um Überlagerungen mit der Halswirbelsäule zu vermeiden, sind Kopf und Hals in Richtung des Widerrists zu strecken.
Zur Verringerung der Streustrahlung ist eine Bucky-Blende oder eine Kassette mit stehendem Raster erforderlich.
Der Zentralstrahl sollte die Mitte des Gelenks in Höhe des Tuberculum majus treffen und im rechten Winkel auf die Kassette einfallen.

Fig. 65 Positioning of shoulder joint, recumbent. Mediolateral.

The leg to be examined (the lower one) should be extended far forward, the free one should be pulled far caudally and secured. In order to avoid overlaying of the cervical spine, the head and neck should be extended dorsally.
A Bucky diaphragm or a cassette with a stationary grid will be necessary to reduce scattered radiation.
The central beam should strike the center of the joint at the level of the tuberculum majus and fall at right angles to the cassette.

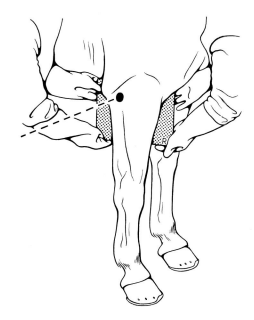

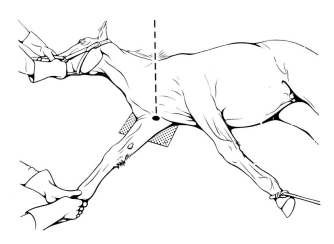

Abb. 66 Lagerung zur Aufnahme des Ellbogengelenks, stehend. Latero-medial.

Um die Kassette zwischen Gliedmaße und Brustkorb ausreichend hoch lagern zu können, sind zwei Hilfspersonen erforderlich. Die Kassette ist so hoch zu drücken, daß der obere Kassettenrand fingerbreit oberhalb des Ellbogenhöckers zu liegen kommt.
Zur Verringerung der Streustrahlung ist eine Kassette mit stehendem Raster erforderlich.
Der Zentralstrahl sollte die Mitte der Außenseite der Extremität fingerbreit proximal des lateralen Bandhöckers des Radius treffen und im rechten Winkel auf die Kassette einfallen.

Fig. 66 Positioning of elbow joint, standing. Lateromedial.

Two assistants are required to hold the cassette sufficiently high enough between the chest and the leg. The cassette must be placed high enough to ensure its upper edge being one fingerwidth above the olecranon.
A stationary grid will be necessary to reduce scattered radiation.
The central beam should strike the center of the lateral aspect of the leg one handwidth distal to the olecranon tuberosity and fall at right angles to the cassette.

Abb. 67 Lagerung zur Aufnahme des Ellbogengelenks, liegend. Medio-lateral.

Die zu untersuchende (untenliegende) Gliedmaße ist so weit nach vorn und die obenliegende so weit nach hinten zu ziehen, bis der Ellbogenhöcker ohne Überlagerung durch die Unterbrust dargestellt ist. Die Lagerung kann durch geringes Anheben der obenliegenden Gliedmaße erleichtert werden.
Zur Verringerung der Streustrahlung ist eine Bucky-Blende oder eine Kassette mit stehendem Raster zu verwenden.
Der Zentralstrahl sollte die Mitte der Innenseite der Extremität fingerbreit proximal des medialen Bandhöckers des Radius treffen und im rechten Winkel auf die Kassette einfallen.

Fig. 67 Positioning of elbow joint, recumbent. Mediolateral.

The leg to be examined (the lower one) should be pulled as far forward and the free one as far caudally as possible to ensure radiography of the free olecranon without overlaying of the lower chest. The positioning can be facilitated by slight lifting of the upper leg.
The Bucky diaphragm or a cassette with a stationary grid should be used to reduce scattered radiation.
The central beam should strike the center of the medial aspect of the leg at a point situated one handwidth distal to the olecranon tuberosity and fall at right angles to the cassette.

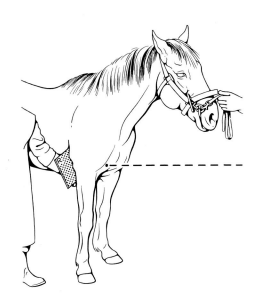

Abb. 68 Lagerung zur Aufnahme des Ellbogengelenks, stehend. Kranio-kaudal.

Die Kassette ist der kaudalen Fläche des Unterarms so anzulegen, daß sich der obere Kassettenrand etwa zweifingerbreit proximal des Tuber olecrani befindet. Dabei ist die Kassette kräftig gegen den Brustkorb zu drücken. Die Kassettenlagerung ist einfacher, wenn die Gliedmaße in leichter Innenrotation belastet oder von einer zweiten Person etwas abduziert werden kann.
Der Zentralstrahl sollte die Mitte der kranialen Fläche des Gelenks fingerbreit proximal des lateralen Bandhöckers des Radius treffen und im rechten Winkel auf die Kassette einfallen.

Fig. 68 Positioning of elbow joint, standing. Craniocaudal.

The cassette should be placed against the caudal surface of the forearm with the upper edge situated approximately two fingerwidths proximal to the olecranon tuberosity. The cassette should be pressed firmly against the chest. The placing of the cassette is facilitated if the limb takes weight in slight inward rotation or if it is held by a second person in a slightly abducted position.
The central beam should strike the middle of the cranial surface of the joint one fingers' width proximal to the lateral tuberosity of the radius and fall at right angles to the cassette.

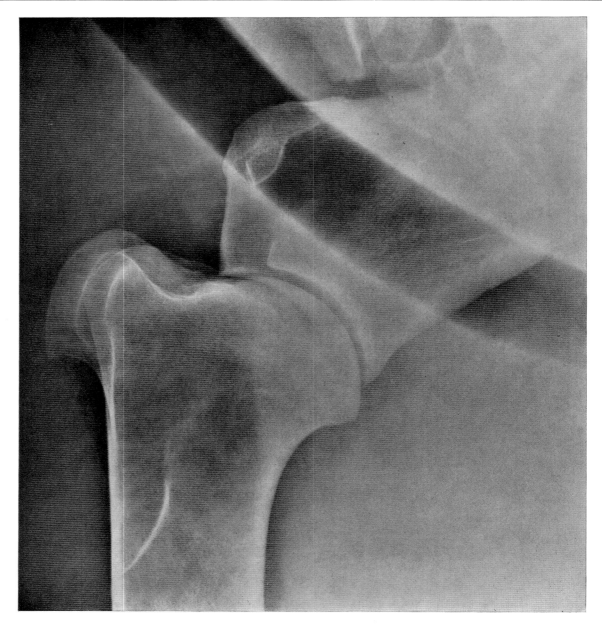

Abb. 69   Rechtes Schultergelenk. Medio-lateral. Warmblut, 13 Jahre.
Bucky-Blende — Feinzeichnende Folie — FFA 100 cm — 90 kV — 85 mAs
Verkleinerung von 30 × 40 cm
Lagerung Abb. 65

Fig. 69   Right shoulder joint. Mediolateral. Light horse, 13 years old.
Bucky diaphragm — High definition screens — FFD 100 cm — 90 kV — 85 mAs
Diminution of 30 × 40 cm
Positioning fig. 65

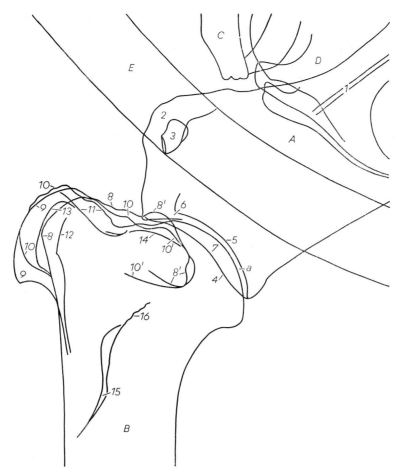

Abb. 70 Röntgenskizze zu Abb. 69   Fig. 70 X-ray sketch to fig. 69

A Scapula;
B Humerus;
C 6. Vertebra cervicalis;
D 7. Vertebra cervicalis;
E Trachea;

a Articulatio humeri;

1 Spina scapulae;
2 Tuberculum supraglenoidale;
3 Processus coracoideus;
4, 5 Cavitas glenoidalis:
4 Lateraler Rand — Lateral border,
5 Medialer Rand — Medial border;
6 Incisura glenoidalis;
7 Caput humeri;
8 Tuberculum majus, Pars cranialis (8) et Pars caudalis (8');

9 Tuberculum intermedium;
10 Tuberculum minus, Pars cranialis (10) et Pars caudalis (10');
11 Orthograph getroffene Kompakta zwischen Caput und Tubercula — Orthographically struck compacta between head and tubercles;
12, 13 Kompaktaschatten, die durch die Konkavität der Sulci intertuberculares lateralis (12) et medialis (13) bedingt sind — Compacta shadows formed by the concavity of the lateral (12) and medial (13) intertubercular grooves;
14 Kompaktaschatten, der durch die Konkavität im Bereich der Aufwölbung der Facies articularis des Caput humeri zum Tuberculum majus, Pars caudalis, entsteht — Compacta shadow formed by the concavity in the area where the articular surface of the humeral head ascends to become continuous with the caudal part of the major tuberosity;
15 Tuberositas deltoidea;
16 Linea musculi tricipitis.

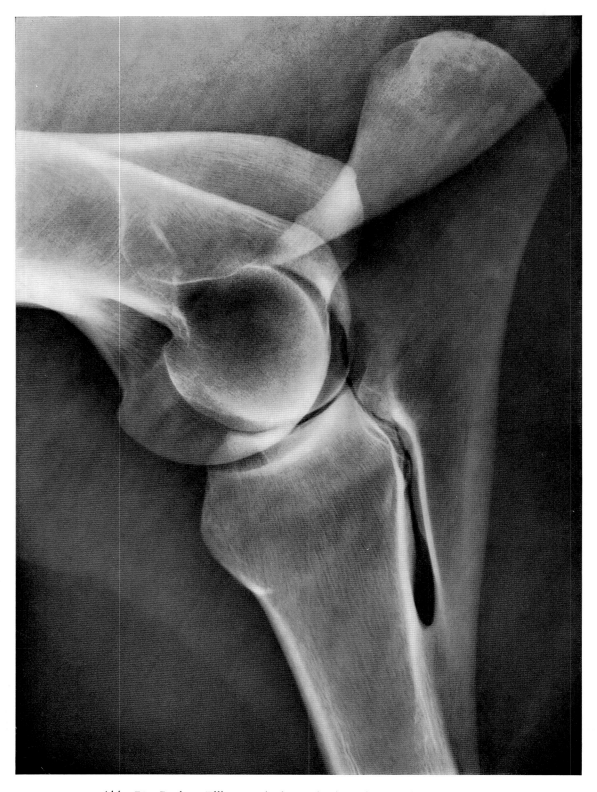

Abb. 71   Rechtes Ellbogengelenk. Medio-lateral. Warmblut, 20 Jahre.
Bucky-Blende — Feinzeichnende Folie — FFA 100 cm — 90 kV — 10 mAs
Ausschnitt und Verkleinerung von 30 × 40 cm
Lagerung Abb. 67

Fig. 71   Right elbow joint. Mediolateral. Light horse, 20 years old.
Bucky diaphragm — High definition screens — FFD 100 cm — 90 kV — 10 mAs
Section and diminution of 30 × 40 cm
Positioning fig. 67

A   Humerus;
B   Radius;
C   Ulna;

a   Articulatio cubiti;
b   Articulatio radioulnaris proximalis;

1, 2   Condylus humeri:
1   Capitulum humeri,
2   Trochlea humeri;
1′ 2′   Facies articularis in der Fossa olecrani — Facies articularis in the olecranon fossa:

1′   Kaudolateraler Rand — Caudolateral border,
2′   Kaudomedialer Rand — Caudomedial border;
3   Kompaktaschatten, der sich aus der Konkavität der Führungsrinne zwischen 1 und 2 ergibt — Compacta shadow formed by the concavity of the groove between 1 and 2;
4   Sagittalkamm am Capitulum humeri — Sagittal crest on the humeral capitulum;
5   Epicondylus lateralis;
6   Crista epicondyli lateralis;
7   Epicondylus medialis;
8   Fossa olecrani, Grund — Fossa olecrani, floor;

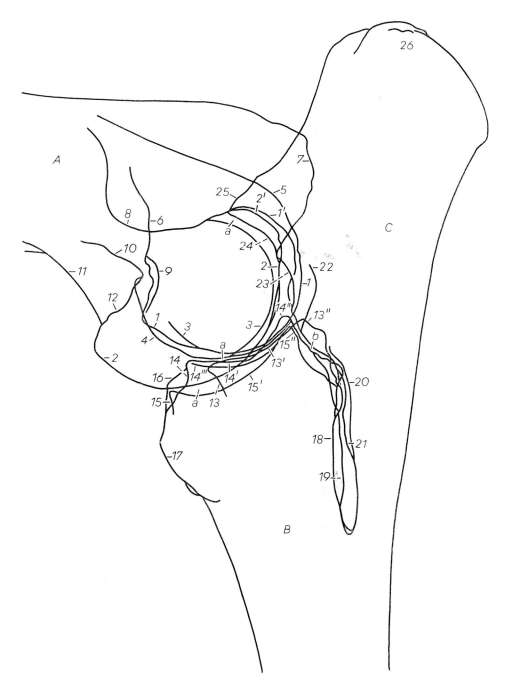

Abb. 72 Röntgenskizze zu Abb. 71   Fig. 72 X-ray sketch to fig. 71

9—11 Fossa radialis:
9 Grund — Floor,
10 Laterale Begrenzung — Lateral limit,
11 Mediale Begrenzung — Medial limit;
12 Facies articularis condyli humeri, proximokranialer Rand — Facies articularis condyli humeri, craniodorsal border;
13—13″ Caput radii, lateraler Abschnitt — Caput radii, lateral part:
13 Kraniale Begrenzung — Cranial border,
13′ Proximale Begrenzung = laterale Hälfte der lateralen Fovea capitis radii — Dorsal border = lateral part of the lateral articular surface,
13″ Kaudale Begrenzung = kaudale Begrenzung des lateralen Bandhöckers — Caudal border = caudal border of the lateral tuberosity;
14—14″ Caput radii, mittlerer Abschnitt — Caput radii, middle part:
14 Kraniale Begrenzung — Cranial border,
14′ Proximale Begrenzung — Dorsal border,
14″ Kaudale Begrenzung — Caudal border;
14‴ Kompaktaschatten, der sich aus der Konkavität des mittleren Bereichs der Fovea capitis radii ergibt — Compacta shadow formed by the concavity of the middle part of the fovea capitis radii;
15—15″ Caput radii, medialer Abschnitt — Caput radii, medial part:

15 Kraniale Begrenzung — Cranial border,
15′ Proximale Begrenzung — Dorsal border,
15″ Kaudale Begrenzung — Caudal border;
16 Fovea capitis radii, proximokraniale Grenze — Fovea capitis radii, craniodorsal border;
17 Tuberositas radii;
18 Margo lateralis radii;
19 Margo medialis radii;
20 Margo lateralis ulnae;
21 Margo medialis ulnae;
22 Processus coronoideus lateralis, zur Incisura trochlearis aufstrebender Rand — Processus coronoideus lateralis, border ascending towards the trochlear incisure;
23 Processus coronoideus medialis, zur Incisura trochlearis aufstrebender Rand — Processus coronoideus medialis, border ascending to the trochlear incisure;
24 Incisura trochlearis, kranialer Rand — Incisura trochlearis, cranial border;
25 Processus anconaeus;
26 Tuber olecrani.

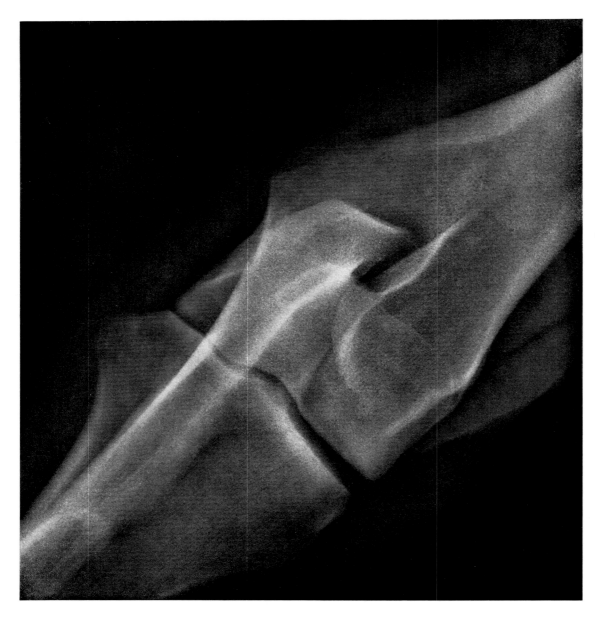

Abb. 73   Rechtes Ellbogengelenk. Kranio-
kaudal. Warmblut, 16 Jahre.
Bucky-Blende — Feinzeichnende Folie
FFA 100 cm — 70 kV — 50 mAs
Verkleinerung von 24 × 30 cm
Lagerung Abb. 68

Fig. 73   Right elbow joint. Craniocaudal.
Light horse, 16 years old.
Bucky diaphragm — High definition screens
FFD 100 cm — 70 kV — 50 mAs
Diminution of 24 × 30 cm
Positioning fig. 68

A Humerus;
B Radius;
C Ulna;

a Articulatio cubiti;

Am Humerus — On the humerus:

1–1″ Condylus humeri:
1′ Kraniale Begrenzung — Cranial border,
1″ Kaudale Begrenzung an der Trochlea —
Caudal border of the trochlea;
2 Laterale Bandgrube — Lateral depression
for ligamentous attachment;
3 Lateraler Bandhöcker — Lateral eminence
for ligamentous attachment;
4 Crista epicondyli lateralis;
5 Epicondylus lateralis;
6 Mediale Bandgrube — Medial depression
for ligamentous attachment;
7 Medialer Bandhöcker — Medial eminence
for ligamentous attachment;
8 Epicondylus medialis;
9, 9′ Fossa olecrani:
9 Orthograph getroffener Abschnitt der
medialen Begrenzung — Orthographically
struck part of the medial limit,
9′ Laterale Begrenzung — Lateral limit;

Am Radius — On the radius:

10–10″ Fovea capitis radii:
10 Verschattung, die sich aus ihrer Konkavität ergibt — Shadow formed by its concavity,

10′ Kraniale Begrenzung — Cranial border,
10″ Kaudale Begrenzung, nur abschnittsweise
identifizierbar — Caudal border, only partly seen;
11 Lateraler Bandhöcker — Lateral eminence
for ligamentous attachment;
12 Medialer Bandhöcker — Medial eminence
for ligamentous attachment;

An der Ulna — On the ulna:

13–13‴ Tuber olecrani:
13′ Kranialer Abschnitt — Cranial part,
13″ Kaudaler Abschnitt — Caudal part,
13‴ Ortograph getroffene Kompakta im Bereich des kaudalen Abschnitts — Orthographically struck compacta in the caudal
area;
14, 15 Olecranon:
14 Laterale Begrenzung — Lateral border,
15 Mediale Begrenzung — Medial border;
16, 17 Incisura trochlearis:
16 Lateraler Rand — Lateral border,
17 Medialer Rand — Medial border;
18 Processus coronoideus lateralis;
19 Processus coronoideus medialis;
20 Margo lateralis ulnae;
21 Margo medialis ulnae.

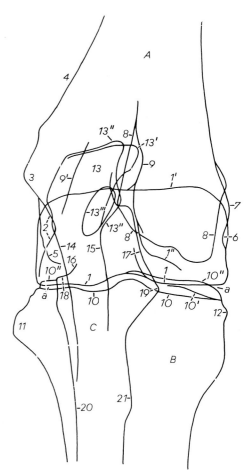

Abb. 74   Röntgenskizze zu Abb. 73

Fig. 74   X-ray sketch to fig. 73

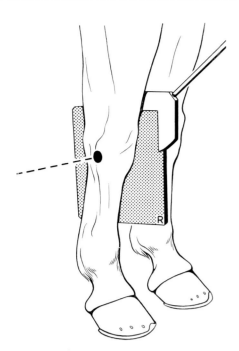

Abb. 75 Lagerung zur Aufnahme des Karpalgelenks. Latero-medial.
Wegen der relativ kleinen Auflagefläche ist eine Verkantung der Kassette leicht möglich. Dem ist durch eine sorgfältige Ausblendung und Einstellung vorzubeugen.
Zur Verringerung der Streustrahlung ist eine Bucky-Blende oder eine Kassette mit stehendem Raster erforderlich.
Der Zentralstrahl sollte auf die Mitte des mittleren (horizontalen) Gelenkspalts treffen und im rechten Winkel auf die Kassette einfallen.

Fig. 75 Positioning of carpal joint. Lateromedial.
In view of the relatively small contact surface, tilting of the cassette can easily occur. Careful setting of the shutter and proper positioning, however, will obviate this problem.
A Bucky diaphragm or a cassette with a stationary grid will be necessary to reduce scattered radiation.
The central beam should strike the center of the middle (horizontal) articular space and fall at right angles to the cassette.

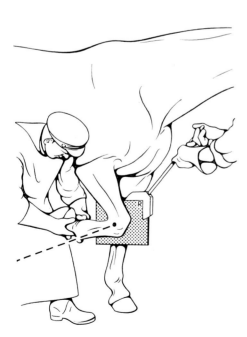

Abb. 76 Lagerung zur Aufnahme des Karpalgelenks, gebeugt. Latero-medial.
Zur Beurteilung des mittleren (horizontalen) Gelenks kann die Aufnahme bei gebeugtem Karpus zweckmäßig sein. Die senkrecht gehaltene Kassette wird dem Karpus und Unterarm angelegt.
Zur Verringerung der Streustrahlung ist eine Bucky-Blende oder eine Kassette mit stehendem Raster erforderlich.
Der Zentralstrahl sollte die Mitte der Gelenkaußenfläche in Höhe des mittleren Gelenkspalts treffen und im rechten Winkel auf die Kassette einfallen.

Fig. 76 Positioning of carpal joint, flexed. Lateromedial.
In evaluating the middle (horizontal) joint, radiography of the flexed carpus is recommended. The cassette should be held perpendicularly and placed against the carpus and forearm.
A Bucky diaphragm or a cassette with a stationary grid will be necessary to reduce scattered radiation.
The central beam should strike the center of the lateral surface of the joint on a level of the middle articular space and fall at right angles to the cassette.

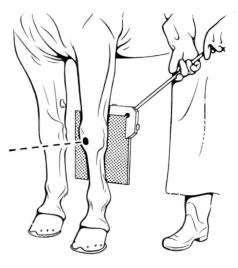

Abb. 77 Lagerung zur Aufnahme des Karpalgelenks. Dorso-palmar.
Beim Ausblenden und der Wahl des Filmformats ist darauf zu achten, daß ein genügend großer Abschnitt des Radius und des Metakarpus abgebildet werden. Um die Folienunschärfe gering zu halten, sollte unter Inkaufnahme einer längeren Belichtungszeit eine feinzeichnende Folie verwendet werden. Schwierig ist die korrekte Lagerung der Kassette, weil sie einer nur relativ kleinen Fläche aufliegt. Durch sorgfältige Einstellung sind Verkantungen zu vermeiden.
Zur Verringerung der Streustrahlung ist eine Bucky-Blende oder eine Kassette mit stehendem Raster erforderlich.
Der Zentralstrahl sollte die Mitte des mittleren (horizontalen) Gelenkspalts treffen und im rechten Winkel auf die Kassette einfallen.

Fig. 77 Positioning of carpal joint. Dorsopalmar.
In selecting the size of the film and in setting the shutter, care must be exercised to reproduce sufficiently large segments of the radius and the metacarpus. In order to keep the loss of fine details at a minimum, high definition screens should be used at the expense of longer exposure time. The proper placing of the cassette is difficult since it makes contact with only a relatively small surface. However, by careful positioning, tilting of the cassette can be avoided.
A Bucky diaphragm or a cassette with a stationary grid will be necessary to reduce scattered radiation.
The central beam should strike the center of the middle (horizontal) articular space and fall at right angles to the cassette.

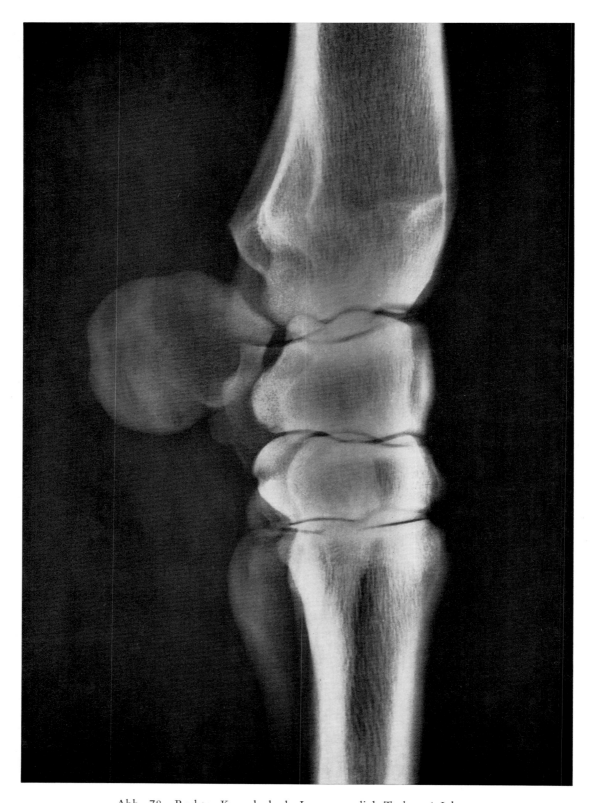

Abb. 78 Rechtes Karpalgelenk. Latero-medial. Traber, 6 Jahre.
Bucky-Blende — Feinzeichnende Folie — FFA 110 cm — 60 kV — 63 mAs
Originalgröße (Ausschnitt aus 24 × 30 cm)
Lagerung Abb. 75

Fig. 78 Right carpal joint. Lateromedial. Trotter, 6 years old.
Bucky diaphragm — High definition screens — FFD 110 cm — 60 kV — 63 mAs
Original size (section of 24 × 30 cm)
Positioning fig. 75

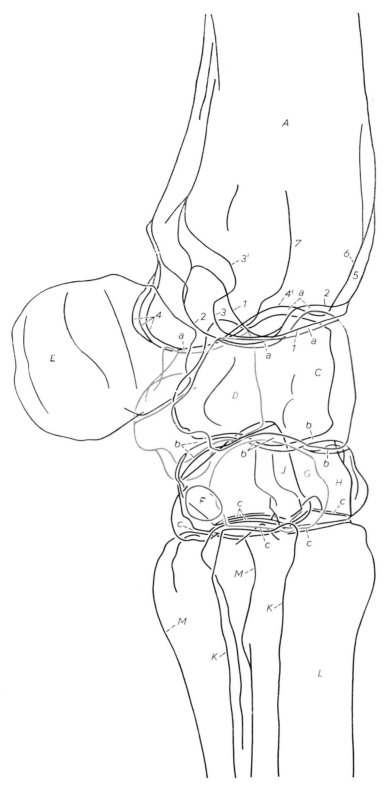

Abb. 79** Röntgenskizze zu Abb. 78   Fig. 79** X-ray sketch to fig. 78

A   Radius;
B   Os carpi radiale;
C   Os carpi intermedium;
D   Os carpi ulnare;
E   Os carpi accessorium;
F   Os carpale I;
G   Os carpale II;
H   Os carpale III;
J   Os carpale IV;
K   Os metacarpale II;
L   Os metacarpale III;
M   Os metacarpale IV;

a   Articulatio antebrachiocarpea;
b   Articulatio mediocarpea;
c   Articulationes carpometacarpeae;

An der Trochlea radii — On the trochlea radii:

1, 2 Medialer Gelenkflächenabschnitt — Medial part of the articular surface:

1   Mediale Begrenzung — Medial border,
2   Laterale Begrenzung — Lateral (axial) border;
3   Mittlerer Gelenkflächenabschnitt, kaudale Begrenzung — Middle facet of the articular surface, caudal border;
3′ Tiefste Stelle der Grube proximal des mittleren Gelenkflächenabschnitts — Floor of the groove proximal to the middle facet of the articular surface;
4, 4′ Lateraler Gelenkflächenabschnitt — Lateral part of the articular surface:
4   Kaudale Begrenzung — Caudal border,
4′ Kraniale Begrenzung — Cranial border;
5, 6 Sehnenrinne des M. extensor carpi radialis — Groove for the tendon of m. extensor carpi radialis:
5   Mediale Begrenzung — Medial border,
6   Laterale Begrenzung — Lateral border;
7   Sehnenrinne des M. extensor digitalis communis, laterale Begrenzung — Groove for the tendon of m. extensor digitalis communis, lateral border.

62

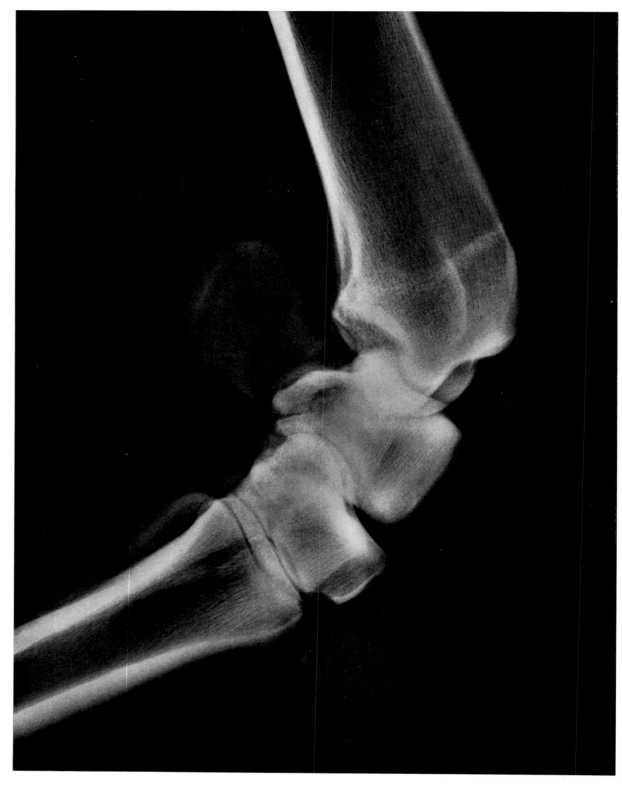

Abb. 80 Rechtes Karpalgelenk, gebeugt. Latero-medial. Traber, 5 Jahre.
Bucky-Blende — Feinzeichnende Folie — FFA 110 cm — 62 kV — 30 mAs
Originalgröße (Ausschnitt aus 24 × 30 cm)
Lagerung Abb. 76

Fig. 80 Right carpal joint, flexed. Lateromedial. Trotter, 5 years old.
Bucky diaphragm — High definition screens — FFD 110 cm — 62 kV — 30 mAs
Original size (section of 24 × 30 cm)
Positioning fig. 76

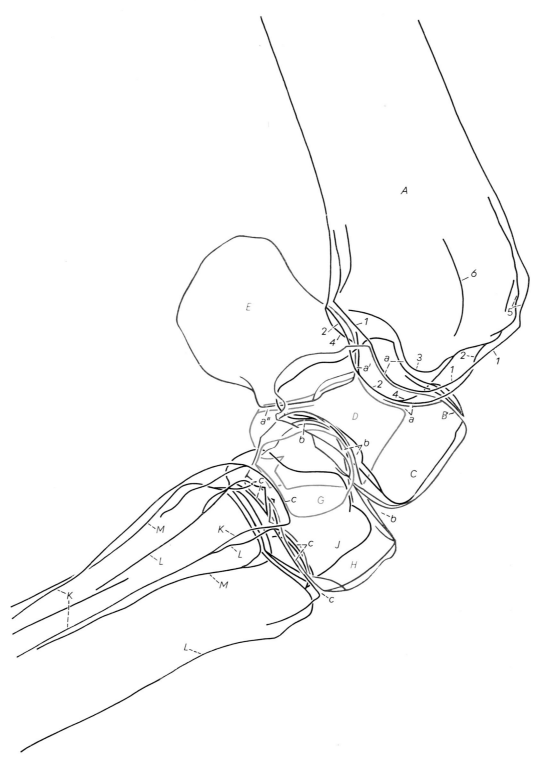

Abb. 81** Röntgenskizze zu Abb. 80   Fig. 81** X-ray sketch to fig. 80

A   Radius;
B   Os carpi radiale;
C   Os carpi intermedium;
D   Os carpi ulnare;
E   Os carpi accessorium;
    (Os carpale I bei diesem Pferd nicht ausgebildet — Os carpale I not
    developed in this horse)
G   Os carpale II;
H   Os carpale III;
J   Os carpale IV;
K   Os metacarpale II;
L   Os metacarpale III;
M   Os metacarpale IV;

a   Articulatio antebrachiocarpea;
a' Gelenkspalte zwischen Radius und Os carpi accessorium — Joint
    space between radius and accessory carpal bone;
a'' Gelenkspalte zwischen Os carpi accessorium und Os carpi ulnare —
    Joint space between accessory and ulnar carpal bones;

b   Articulatio mediocarpea;
c   Articulationes carpometacarpeae;

An der Trochlea radii — On the trochlea radii:

1, 2 Medialer Gelenkflächenabschnitt — Medial facet of the articular
     surface:
1   Mediale Begrenzung — Medial border,
2   Laterale Begrenzung — Lateral (axial) border;
3   Mittlerer Gelenkflächenabschnitt — Middle facet of the articular
     surface;
4   Begrenzung des lateralen Gelenkflächenabschnitts — Border of the
     lateral facet of the articular surface;
5   Begrenzung der Sehnenrinne des M. extensor carpi radialis — Border
     of the groove for the tendon of m. extensor carpi radialis;
6   Begrenzung der Sehnenrinne des M. extensor digitalis communis —
     Border of the groove for the tendon of m. extensor digitalis
     communis.

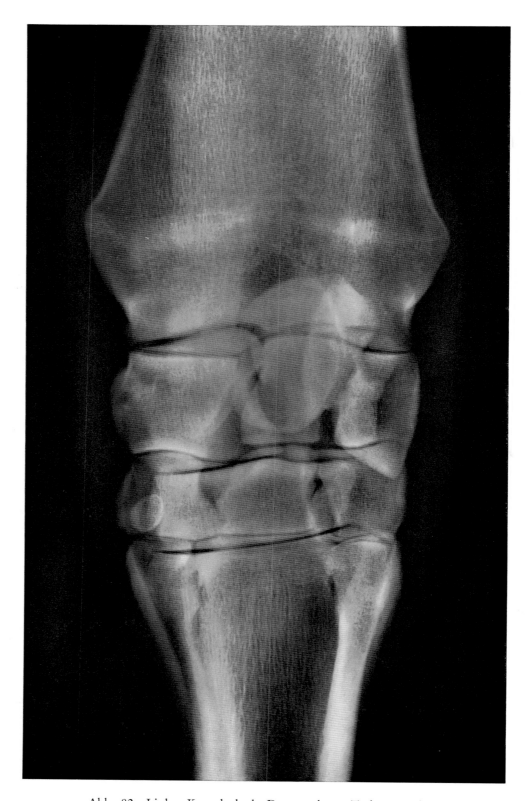

Abb. 82 Linkes Karpalgelenk. Dorso-palmar. Traber, 6 Jahre.
Bucky-Blende — Feinzeichnende Folie — FFA 110 cm — 62 kV — 30 mAs
Originalgröße (Ausschnitt aus 24 × 30 cm)
Lagerung Abb. 77

Fig. 82 Left carpal joint. Dorsopalmar. Trotter, 6 years old.
Bucky diaphragm — High definition screens — FFD 110 cm — 62 kV — 30 mAs
Original size (section of 24 × 30 cm)
Positioning fig. 77

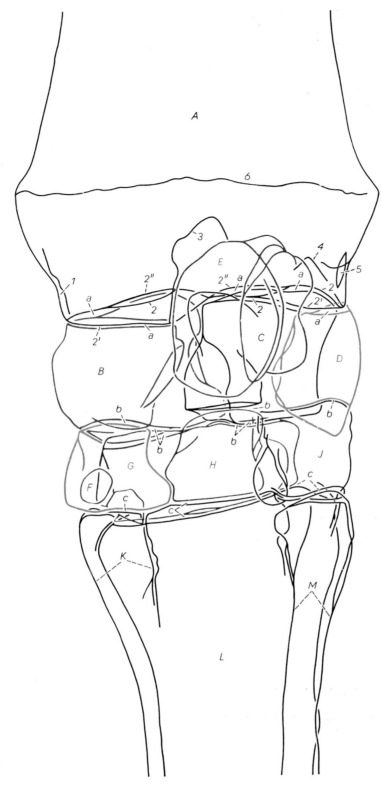

Abb. 83** Röntgenskizze zu Abb. 82   Fig. 83** X-ray sketch to fig. 82

A   Radius;
B   Os carpi radiale;
C   Os carpi intermedium;
D   Os carpi ulnare;
E   Os carpi accessorium;
F   Os carpale I;
G   Os carpale II;
H   Os carpale III;
J   Os carpale IV;
K   Os metacarpale II;
L   Os metacarpale III;
M   Os metacarpale IV;

a   Articulatio antebrachiocarpea;
b   Articulatio mediocarpea;
c   Articulationes carpometacarpeae;

An der Trochlea radii — On the trochlea radii:

1   Bandgrube am Processus styloideus medialis — Depression on the medial styloid process for ligamentous attachment;
2—4 Trochlea radii:
2   Dorsaler Rand — Dorsal border,
2'   Distale Begrenzung — Distal border,
2'' Die aus der Konkavität resultierende Begrenzung — Border formed by the concavity,
3   Kaudale Begrenzung des mittleren Gelenkflächenabschnitts — Caudal border of the middle facet of the articular surface,
4   Kaudale Begrenzung des lateralen Gelenkflächenabschnitts — Caudal border of the lateral facet of the articular surface;
5   Bandgrube am Processus styloideus lateralis — Depression on the lateral styloid process for ligamentous attachment;
6   Crista transversa.

Lagerung der Kassette zur Aufnahme der Griffelbeine.
Zur Aufnahme der Griffelbeine ergeben sich die in den Abbildungen 84 und 85 dargestellten Möglichkeiten zur Lagerung der Kassette und die Einstellungen des Strahlengangs.
Der Zentralstrahl sollte das Griffelbein im mittleren Drittel treffen und im rechten Winkel auf die Kassette einfallen.

Positioning of the cassette for the splint bones.
In radiographing the splint bones, various possibilities of placing the cassette and focusing the beam are shown in figs. 84 and 85.
The central beam should strike the splint bone in the middle third and fall at right angles to the cassette.

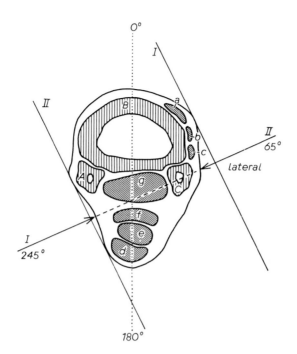

Abb. 84   Lagerung der Kassette zur Darstellung des lateralen Griffelbeins der rechten Schultergliedmaße.

Fig. 84   Positioning of the cassette for the lateral splint bone of the right thoracic limb.

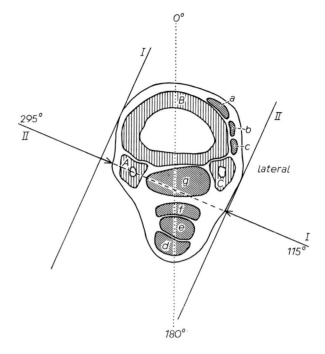

Abb. 85   Lagerung der Kassette zur Darstellung des medialen Griffelbeins der rechten Schultergliedmaße.

Fig. 85   Positioning of the cassette for the medial splint bone of the right thoracic limb.

A   Os metacarpale II;
B   Os metacarpale III;
C   Os metacarpale IV;

a   Sehne des M. extensor digitalis communis — Tendon of m. extensor digitalis communis;
b   Lateraler Teil des M. extensor digitalis communis (Phillipsscher Muskel) — Radial head of m. extensor digitalis communis (muscle of Phillips);

c   Sehne des M. extensor digitalis lateralis — Tendon of m. extensor digitalis lateralis;
d   Sehne des M. flexor digitalis superficialis — Tendon of m. flexor digitalis superficialis;
e   Sehne des M. flexor digitalis profundus — Tendon of m. flexor digitalis profundus,
f   Sehniger Unterstützungsschenkel, Ligamentum accessorium — Carpal check ligament, accessory ligament;
g   M. interosseus medius.

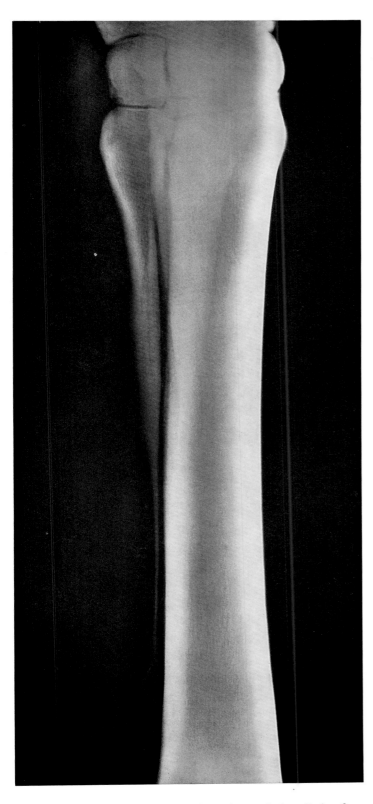

Abb. 86 Mediales Griffelbein der rechten Schultergliedmaße.
Traber, 3 Jahre.
Feinzeichnende Folie — FFA 100 cm — 50 kV — 23 mAs
Verkleinerung von 24 × 30 cm
Lagerung Abb. 85

Fig. 86 Medial splint bone of right thoracic limb. Trotter, 3 years old.
High definition screens — FFD 100 cm — 50 kV — 23 mAs
Diminution of 24 × 30 cm
Positioning fig. 85

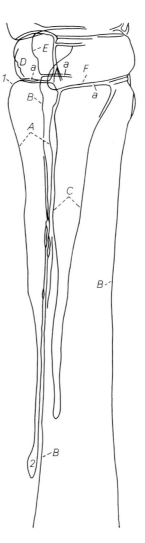

Abb. 87 Röntgenskizze zu Abb. 86
Fig. 87 X-ray sketch to fig. 86

A   Os metacarpale II;
B   Os metacarpale III;
C   Os metacarpale IV;
D   Os carpale II;
E   Os carpale III;
F   Os carpale IV;

a   Articulationes carpometacarpeae;

1   Griffelbeinköpfchen, Basis des Os metacarpale II — Base of the medial splint bone;
2   Griffelbeinknöpfchen, Caput-Rudiment des Os metacarpale II — Button of the medial splint bone.

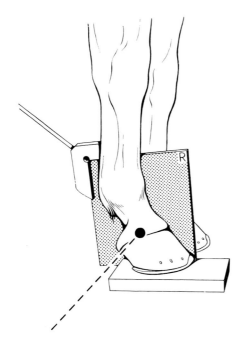

Abb. 88   Lagerung zur Aufnahme des Fessel-, Kron- und Hufgelenks.
Latero-medial.

Bei einer Zehenübersichtsaufnahme sollte der Zentralstrahl die Mitte der
Gliedmaßenaußenseite in Höhe des Krongelenks treffen und im rechten
Winkel auf die Kassette einfallen.
Zur Aufnahme des Fesselgelenks sollte der Zentralstrahl in Höhe der
distalen Gleichbeinkante die Mitte der Gelenkaußenfläche treffen und im
rechten Winkel auf die Kassette einfallen.
Um den distalen Zehenbereich bei horizontalem Strahlengang aufnehmen
zu können, ist die zu untersuchende Gliedmaße auf einen etwa 5 cm starken Holzklotz so zu stellen, daß der mediale Tragrand an der Kante des
Holzklotzes steht. Bei unruhigen Pferden oder wenn die aufzunehmende
Gliedmaße wegen der Höherstellung nicht ausreichend belastet wird,
empfiehlt es sich, die andere Schultergliedmaße wie zum Beschlag hochheben zu lassen.
Zur Aufnahme des Hufgelenks bzw. des Hufbeins sollte der Zentralstrahl die weiteste Stelle des Hufes in Höhe des Kronrands treffen und
im rechten Winkel auf die Kassette einfallen.

Fig. 88   Positioning of the fetlock, pastern, and coffin joints.
Lateromedial.

In routine radiography of the digit, the central beam should strike the
center of the extremity on a level of the pastern joint and fall at right
angles to the cassette.
In radiographing the fetlock joint, the central beam should strike the
center of the joint from the outside on a level of the distal border of the
sesamoid bone and fall at right angles to the cassette.
In radiographing the distal digital region with a horizontal beam, it is
necessary to place the extremity upon a wooden block, approximately
5 cm thick. The medial border of the hoof should rest upon the edge of
the block. In restless horses, or when the leg to be examined does not
bear sufficient weight, the opposite hoof should be lifted and held up.
In radiographing the coffin joint or the distal phalanx, the central beam
should strike the farthest point of the hoof at the level of the coronary
border and fall at right angles to the cassette.

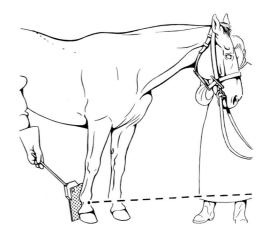

Abb. 89   Lagerung zur Aufnahme der Zehe. Dorso-palmar.

Zur Aufnahme von Fessel- und Kronbein und zur Aufnahme des Krongelenks wird die Kassette dem Fesselkopf und dem Ballen angelegt.
Der Zentralstrahl sollte abhängig von der Fragestellung das Fesselbein in
der Medianebene in halber Höhe (Übersichtsaufnahme) bzw. das Krongelenk in der Mitte treffen und im rechten Winkel auf die Kassette einfallen.
Zur Aufnahme des Fesselgelenks wird die Kassette senkrecht hinter den
Fesselkopf gelagert. Der Zentralstrahl sollte die Mitte der Gliedmaßenvorderfläche in Höhe der distalen Gleichbeinkante treffen und im rechten
Winkel auf die Kassette einfallen.

Fig. 89   Positioning of digit. Dorsopalmar.

In radiographing the proximal and middle phalanges as well as the
pastern joint, the cassette should be placed against the fetlock joint and
the bulbs of the hoof.
Depending on the case in question, the central beam should strike the
axis of the proximal phalanx at the middle of its length (routine radiograph) and the center of the pastern joint respectively and fall at right
angles to the cassette.
In radiographing the fetlock joint, the cassette is placed perpendicularly
behind the joint. The central beam should strike the center of the dorsal
surface of the digit on a level of the distal border of the sesamoid bone
and fall at right angles to the cassette.

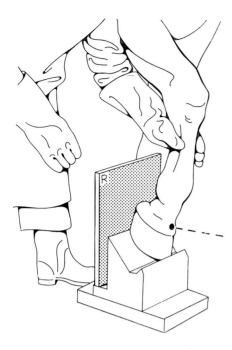

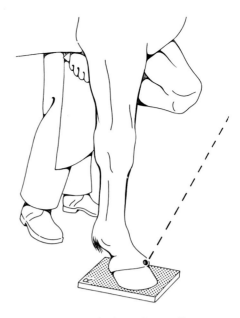

Abb. 91   Lagerung zur Aufnahme des Hufbeins. Dorso-palmar.

Um eine optimale Aufnahme zu erhalten und vor allem um einer falschen Interpretation vorzubeugen, sind vor der röntgenologischen Untersuchung das Hufeisen abzunehmen und der Huf sorgfältig auszuschneiden. Dabei ist besonders auf die Revision der Strahlfurchen (Schmutz entfernen, Abrunden der Furchen) zu achten. Um einer unterschiedlichen Strahlenabsorption durch die Sohle vorzubeugen, wird die Sohlenfläche unmittelbar vor der Untersuchung mit grüner Seife ausgefüllt (auf die Strahlfurchen achten!). Nach Fertigstellung der Aufnahme ist die Seife wieder zu entfernen.

Zur Aufnahme des Hufbeins bei belasteter Gliedmaße ist ein Kassettenschutz erforderlich. Bewährt hat sich eine Plastikbrücke. Um das Ausblenden zu erleichtern und um die Kassette gegebenenfalls erst nach der korrekten Lagerung des Hufes unterlegen oder auswechseln zu können, sollten Höhe und Breite der Brücke dem Kassettenformat entsprechen.

Zur Aufnahme des Hufbeins sollte der Zentralstrahl den distalen Rand des Kronwulstes in der Mitte der dorsalen Fläche treffen und in einem Winkel von 60° auf die Kassette einfallen.

Zur Aufnahme des Strahlbeins sollte der Zentralstrahl den Kronwulst in der Medianen treffen und in einem Winkel von 65° — zur Darstellung des proximalen Strahlbeinrands im Winkel von 45° — auf die Kassette einfallen.

Abb. 90   Lagerung zur Aufnahme des Strahlbeins. Dorso-palmar.

Zur Aufnahme des Strahl- und Hufbeins bei entlasteter Gliedmaße hat sich der abgebildete Holzblock bewährt.

Vor der Röntgenuntersuchung sollten das Hufeisen abgenommen und der Huf sorgfältig ausgeschnitten werden. Dabei ist besonders auf die Revision der Strahlfurchen zu achten. Um eine gleichmäßige Strahlenabsorption durch die Sohle zu erhalten, ist die Sohlenfläche vor der Lagerung zur Aufnahme mit grüner Seife auszufüllen (auf Strahlfurchen achten!). Die Seife ist nach der Röntgenuntersuchung wieder zu entfernen.

Bei dieser Lagerung befindet sich die Sohle in einem Winkel von 45° zu der Kassette. Das Fesselbein sollte annähernd senkrecht stehen.

Zur Verringerung der Streustrahlung ist eine Kassette mit stehendem Raster erforderlich.

Der Zentralstrahl sollte die Krone in der Mitte der Vorderfläche treffen und im rechten Winkel auf die Kassette einfallen.

Fig. 90   Positioning of navicular bone. Dorsopalmar.

In radiography of the distal sesamoid bone and the distal phalanx a wooden block as illustrated is useful.

Before the radiographic examination, the horseshoe should be removed and the hoof properly trimmed. The sulci of the frog should be carefully checked. To ensure even absorption of X-rays by the sole, its surface should be filled with green soap before X-raying. (Mind sulci of the frog!) After radiography the soap should be removed.

In this position the sole is at an angle of 45° to the cassette. The proximal phalanx should be approximately perpendicular.

A stationary grid will be necessary to reduce scattered radiation.

The central beam should strike the coronary border in the center and fall at right angles to the cassette.

Fig. 91   Positioning of coffin bone. Dorsopalmar.

To obtain the desired radiograph and avoid incorrect interpretation, the horseshoe should be removed and the hoof properly trimmed. Special attention must be paid in checking the sulci of the frog (removal of dirt, rounding off the sulci). To prevent uneven absorption of X-rays by the sole, its surface should be filled up with green soap before X-raying. (Mind sulci of the frog!) After the radiograph has been taken, the green soap should be removed.

In radiography of the distal phalanx in the standing position, the cassette must be protected. A plastic bridge is suitable for the purpose. To facilitate setting of the shutter, placing the cassette under the plastic bridge after positioning of the hoof has been accomplished, or exchanging the cassette, the size of the bridge must correspond to that of the cassette.

In radiographing the distal phalanx, the central beam should strike the distal edge of the coronary border at the center on the dorsal surface and fall at an angle of 60° to the cassette.

For radiography of the navicular bone, the central beam should strike the midline of the coronet and fall at an angle of 65° to the cassette, for the proximal border of the navicular bone at an angle of 45° to the cassette.

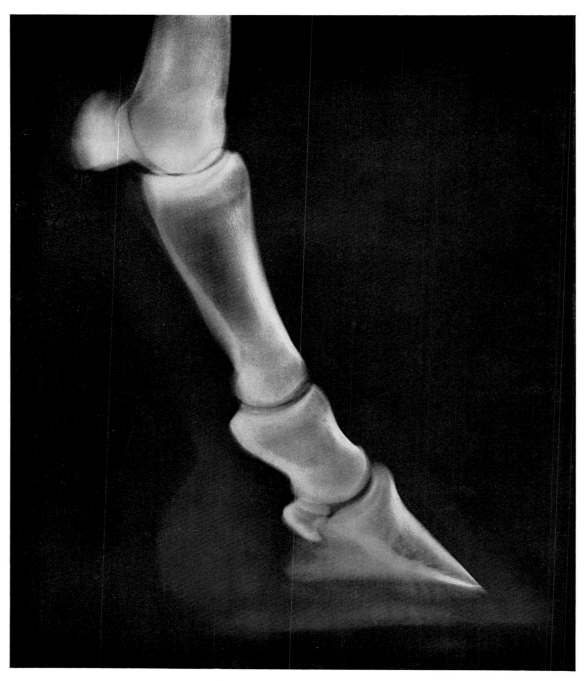

Abb. 92   Zehe der rechten Schultergliedmaße. Latero-medial. Traber, 3 Jahre.
Feinzeichnende Folie — FFA 100 cm — 55 kV — 15 mAs
Verkleinerung von 24 × 30 cm
Lagerung Abb. 88

Fig. 92   Digit of the right thoracic limb. Lateromedial. Trotter, 3 years old.
High definition screens — FFD 100 cm — 55 kV — 15 mAs
Diminution of 24 × 30 cm
Positioning fig. 88

A   Os metacarpale III;
B   Mediales Os sesamoideum proximale — Medial proximal sesamoid bone;
C   Laterales Os sesamoideum proximale — Lateral proximal sesamoid bone;
D   Phalanx proximalis;
E   Phalanx media;
F   Phalanx distalis;
G   Os sesamoideum distale;

a   Articulatio metacarpophalangea;
b   Articulatio interphalangea proximalis manus;
c   Articulatio interphalangea distalis manus;

Am Metakarpus — On the metacarpus:

1   Os metacarpale III, Caput:
2   Sagittalkamm — Sagittal ridge,
3   Lateraler Abschnitt — Lateral part;

An der Phalanx proximalis — On the proximal phalanx:

4, 5   Fovea articularis:
4   Mediale Begrenzung — Medial border,
5   Laterale Begrenzung — Lateral border;
6   Verschattung, die sich aus der Konkavität am Grund der Sagittalrinne ergibt — Shadow formed by the concavity at the base of the sagittal groove;
7   Medialer Bandhöcker — Medial eminence for ligamentous attachment;

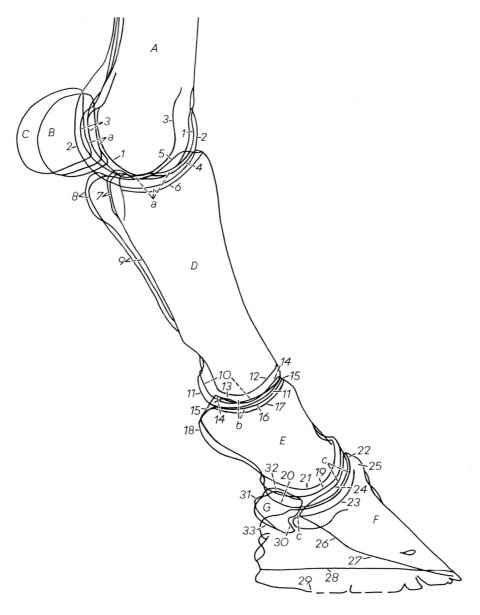

Abb. 93   Röntgenskizze zu Abb. 92

Fig. 93   X-ray sketch to fig. 92

8   Lateraler Bandhöcker — Lateral eminence for ligamentous attachment;

9   Fesselbeinleisten — Ridges on the palmar surface of the proximal phalanx;

10, 11   Trochlea phalangis proximalis:

10   Medialer Abschnitt — Medial part,

11   Lateraler Abschnitt — Lateral part;

12   Verschattung, die sich aus der Konkavität des Sattels vom Caput ergibt — Shadow formed by the concavity of the saddle of the head;

An der Phalanx media — On the middle phalanx:

13   Fovea articularis, mediale Begrenzung — Fovea articularis, medial border;

14   Sagittalkamm — Sagittal ridge;

15   Fovea articularis, laterale Begrenzung — Fovea articularis, lateral border;

16, 17   Verschattungen, die sich aus der Konkavität des medialen (16) bzw. des lateralen (17) Abschnitts der Fovea articularis ergeben — Shadows formed by the concavity of the medial (16) and lateral (17) parts of the articular surface respectively;

18   Kronbeinlehne — Transverse prominence for attachment of scutum medium;

19, 20   Caput phalangis mediae:

19   Medialer Abschnitt — Medial part,

20   Lateraler Abschnitt — Lateral part;

21   Verschattung, die sich aus der Konkavität des Sattels des Caputs ergibt — Shadow formed by the concavity of the saddle of the head;

An der Phalanx distalis — On the distal phalanx:

22, 23   Verschattungen, die sich aus der Konkavität des medialen (22) bzw. lateralen (23) Abschnitts der Fovea articularis ergeben — Shadows formed by the concavity of the medial (22) and lateral (23) parts of the articular surface respectively;

24   Sagittalkamm — Sagittal ridge;

25   Processus extensorius;

26, 27   Orthograph getroffene Abschnitte der Facies flexoria (26) und der Facies solearis (27) — Orthographically struck parts of facies flexoria (26) and facies solearis (27);

28, 29   Margo solearis:

28   Medialer Teil — Medial part,

29   Lateraler Teil — Lateral part;

Am Os sesamoideum distale — On the distal sesamoid bone:

30   Margo distalis;

31   Margo proximalis;

32   Facies articularis;

33   Facies flexoria.

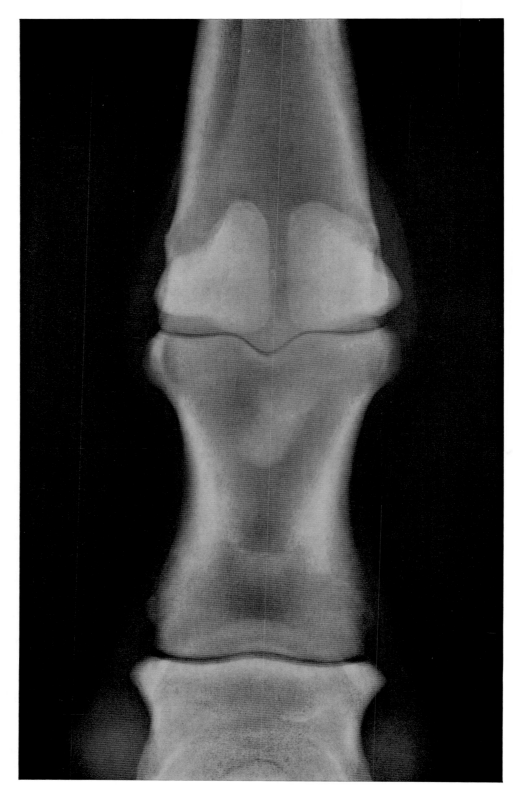

Abb. 94   Fessel- und Krongelenk der rechten Schultergliedmaße.
Dorso-palmar. Warmblut, 3 Jahre.
Feinzeichnende Folie — FFA 100 cm — 60 kV — 25 mAs
Verkleinerung von 24 × 30 cm
Lagerung Abb. 89

Fig. 94   Fetlock and pastern joints of the right thoracic limb.
Dorsopalmar. Light horse, 3 years old.
High definition screens — FFD 100 cm — 60 kV — 25 mAs
Diminution of 24 × 30 cm
Positioning fig. 89

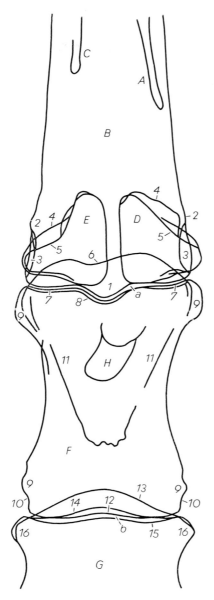

Abb. 95   Röntgenskizze zu Abb. 94   Fig. 95   X-ray sketch to fig. 94

A   Os metacarpale II;
B   Os metacarpale III;
C   Os metacarpale IV;
D   Mediales Os sesamoideum proximale — Medial proximal sesamoid bone;
E   Laterales Os sesamoideum proximale — Lateral proximal sesamoid bone;
F   Phalanx proximalis;
G   Phalanx media;
H   Sporn, Calcar metacarpeum — Ergot;

a   Articulatio metacarpophalangea;
b   Articulatio interphalangea proximalis manus;

Am Metakarpus — On the metacarpus:
1   Trochlea metacarpi, Sagittalkamm — Trochlea metacarpi, sagittal ridge;
2   Bandhöcker — Eminence for ligamentous attachment;
3   Bandgrube — Depression for ligamentous attachment;

An den Ossa sesamoidea proximalia — On the proximal sesamoid bones:
4   Proximopalmarer Randwulst — Proximopalmar marginal thickening;

5   Proximaler Rand der Facies articularis — Proximal border of the articular surface;

An der Phalanx proximalis — On the proximal phalanx:
6, 7   Fovea articularis phalangis proximalis:
6   Dorsaler Rand — Dorsal border,
7   Palmarer Rand — Palmar border;
8   Kompaktaschatten, der durch die Konkavität der Fovea articularis phalangis proximalis bedingt ist — Compacta shadow formed by the concavity of the articular surface of the proximal phalanx;
9   Bandhöcker — Eminence for ligamentous attachment;
10   Bandgrube — Depression for ligamentous attachment;
11   Fesselbeinleisten — Ridges on the palmar surface of the proximal phalanx;
12   Trochlea phalangis proximalis;

An der Phalanx media — On the middle phalanx:
13, 14   Fovea articularis phalangis mediae:
13   Dorsaler Rand — Dorsal border,
14   Palmarer Rand — Palmar border;
15   Kompaktaschatten, der durch die Konkavität der Fovea articularis phalangis mediae bedingt ist — Compacta shadow formed by the concavity of the articular surface of the middle phalanx;
16   Bandhöcker — Eminence for ligamentous attachment.

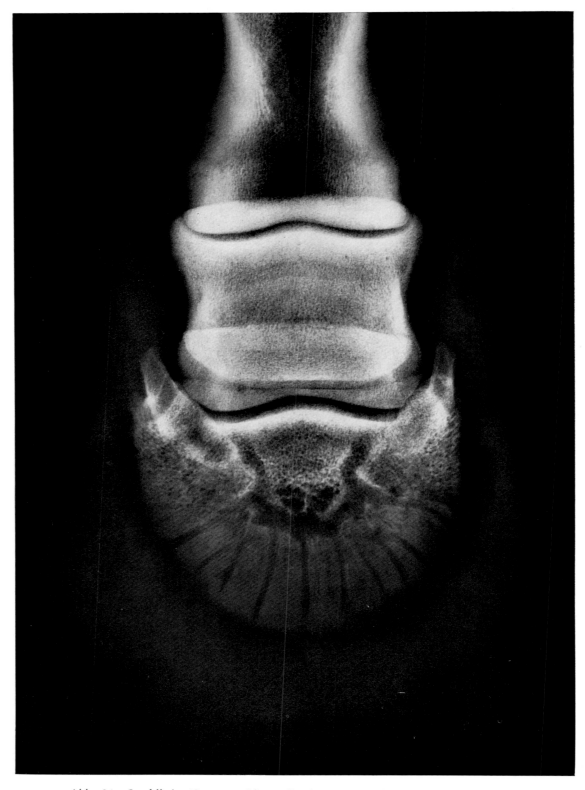

Abb. 96   Strahlbein (Os sesamoideum distale). Dorso-palmar. Warmblut, 3 Jahre
Stehendes Raster — Bucky-Blende — Feinzeichnende Folie — FFA 100 cm — 70 kV — 40 mAs
Originalgröße (Ausschnitt aus 24 × 30 cm)
Lagerung Abb. 90

Fig. 96   Navicular bone (distal sesamoid bone). Dorsopalmar. Light horse, 3 years old.
Stationary grid — Bucky diaphragm — High definition screens — FFD 100 cm — 70 kV — 40 mAs
Original size (section of 24 × 30 cm)
Positioning fig. 90

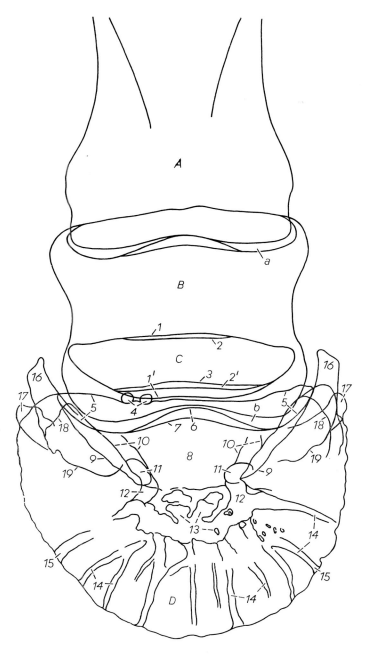

Abb. 97 Röntgenskizze zu Abb. 96   Fig. 97 X-ray sketch to fig. 96

A Phalanx proximalis;
B Phalanx media;
C Os sesamoideum distale;
D Phalanx distalis;

a Articulatio interphalangea proximalis manus;
b Articulatio interphalangea distalis manus;

Am Os sesamoideum distale — On the distal sesamoid bone:

1, 1′ Facies flexoria, proximaler bzw. distaler Rand — Facies flexoria, proximal and distal borders respectively;
2, 2′ Facies articularis, proximaler bzw. distaler Rand — Facies articularis, proximal and distal borders respectively;
3 Unregelmäßig begrenzter Grund der rinnenförmigen Vertiefung am Margo distalis — Irregularly demarcated floor of the groove on the distal border;
4 Orthograph getroffene Gefäße, Aufhellungen gehören nicht zum Os sesamoideum distale — Orthographically struck vessels, rarefactions do not belong to the distal sesamoid bone;

An der Phalanx distalis — On the distal phalanx:

5 Facies articularis;
6 Processus extensorius;
7 Kompaktaschatten, der sich aus der Wölbung der Facies articularis ergibt — Compacta shadow formed by the curvature of the articular surface;
8 Facies flexoria;
9 Linea semilunaris;
10 Begrenzungen der Sulci soleares medialis und lateralis — Borders of the medial and lateral solea grooves respectively;
11 Foramina solearia mediale et laterale;
12 Canalis solearis;
13 Gefäßlöcher im Bereich des Canalis solearis — Vascular foramina in the area of the solea canal;
14, 15 Gefäßkanäle (14) mit Sohlenrandlöchern (15) — Vascular canals (14) with foramina (15) being on or near the distal border;
16, 17 Proximaler und distaler Ast der Processus palmares medialis bzw. lateralis — Proximal and distal parts of the medial and lateral palmar processes respectively;
18 Incisura processus palmaris;
19 Sulcus parietalis.

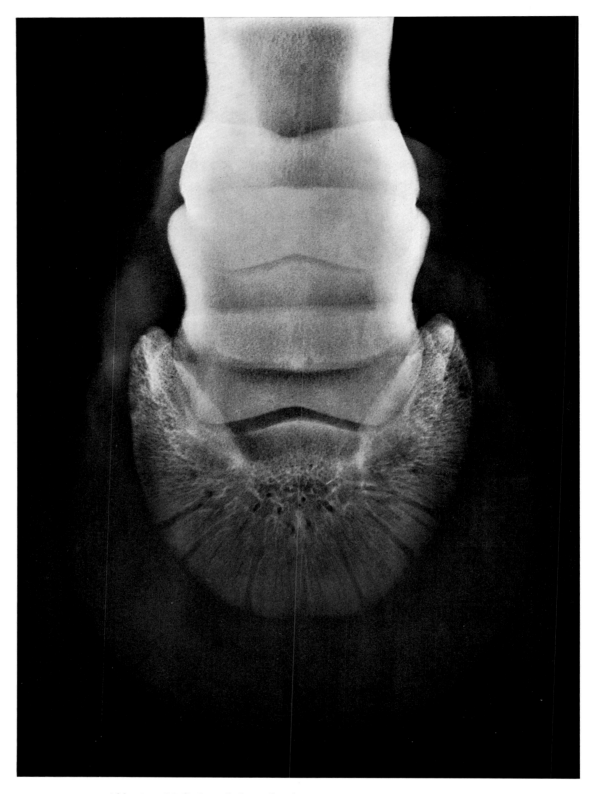

Abb. 98   Hufbein (Phalanx distalis). Dorso-palmar. Traber, 3 Jahre.
Feinzeichnende Folie — FFA 100 cm — 60 kV — 30 mAs
Originalgröße (Ausschnitt aus 24 × 30 cm)
Lagerung Abb. 91

Fig. 98   Coffin bone (distal phalanx). Dorsopalmar. Trotter, 3 years old.
High definition screens — FFD 100 cm — 60 kV — 30 mAs
Original size (section of 24 × 30 cm)
Positioning fig. 91

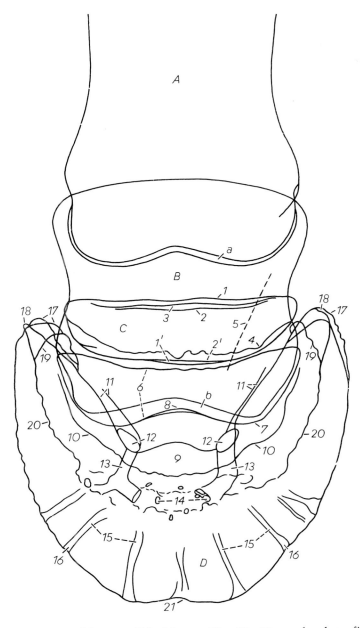

Abb. 99   Röntgenskizze zu Abb. 98   Fig. 99   X-ray sketch to fig. 98

A   Phalanx proximalis;
B   Phalanx media;
C   Os sesamoideum distale;
D   Phalanx distalis;

a   Articulatio interphalangea proximalis manus;
b   Articulatio interphalangea distalis manus;

Am Os sesamoideum distale — On the distal sesamoid bone:

1, 1′ Facies flexoria, proximaler bzw. distaler Rand — Facies flexoria, proximal and distal borders respectively;
2, 2′ Facies articularis, proximaler bzw. distaler Rand — Facies articularis, proximal and distal borders respectively;
3   Grund der rinnenförmigen Vertiefung am Margo proximalis — Floor of the groove on the proximal border;
4   Unregelmäßig begrenzter Grund der rinnenförmigen Vertiefung am Margo distalis — Irregularly demarcated floor of the groove on the distal border;
5   Unzureichend ausgefüllte mediale Strahlfurche — Insufficiently padded medial collateral sulcus of the frog;

An der Phalanx distalis — On the distal phalanx:

6   Facies articularis;
7   Margo coronalis;
8   Processus extensorius;
9   Facies flexoria;
10   Linea semilunaris;
11   Begrenzungen der Sulci soleares medialis bzw. lateralis — Borders of the medial and lateral solea grooves respectively;
12   Foramina solearia mediale et laterale;
13   Canalis solearis;
14   Gefäßlöcher im Bereich des Canalis solearis — Vascular foramina in the area of the solea canal;
15, 16   Gefäßkanäle (15) mit Sohlenrandlöchern (16) — Vascular canals (15) and foramina (16) being on or near the distal border;
17, 18   Proximaler und distaler Ast der Processus palmares medialis bzw. lateralis — Proximal and distal parts of the medial and lateral palmar processes respectively;
19   Incisura processus palmaris;
20   Sulcus parietalis;
21   Crena marginis solearis, Tragrandkerbe — Crena marginis solearis, mid-dorsal notch.

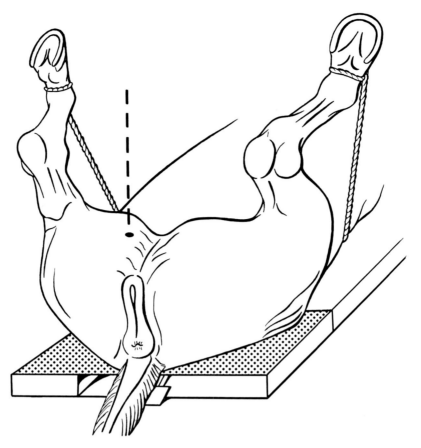

Abb. 100 Lagerung zur Aufnahme des Hüftgelenks. Ventro-dorsal.

Die Darstellung des gesamten Beckens ist wegen seiner Größe nur bei kleinen Tieren möglich. Das zu untersuchende Hüftgelenk sollte auf der Kassette so gelagert sein, daß es in die Mitte des Filmes (30 × 40 cm) projiziert wird.

Zur Reduzierung der Streustrahlung ist eine Kassette mit stehendem Raster oder eine Bucky-Blende erforderlich.

Der Zentralstrahl sollte zweifingerbreit kaudal vom Schambeinkamm und, abhängig von der Größe des Pferdes, bis zu Handbreite neben der Mittellinie auftreffen und im rechten Winkel auf die Kassette einfallen.

Fig. 100 Positioning of hip joint. Ventrodorsal.

Due to its size, radiography of the entire pelvis is possible in small horses only. The hip joint to be examined should be placed exactly at the center of the cassette (30 × 40 cm).

To reduce scattered radiation a stationary grid or a Bucky diaphragm should be used.

The central beam should strike a point two fingerwidths caudally from the pecten of the pubis and, depending on the size of the horse, up to one handwidth laterally from the midline and fall at right angles to the cassette.

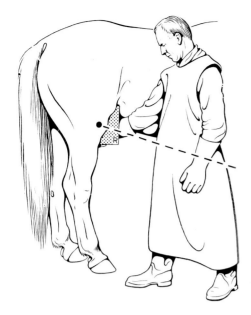

Abb. 101 Lagerung zur Aufnahme des Kniegelenks. Latero-medial.

Am stehenden, gegebenenfalls sedierten Pferd wird die senkrecht gehaltene Kassette dem Kniegelenk medial angelegt und so weit wie möglich nach proximal zwischen Gliedmaße und Bauchdecke gedrückt.
Um eine gute Detailzeichnung zu erhalten, ist, wenn es die Leistung des Röntgengeräts erlaubt, eine feinzeichnende, allenfalls eine mittelverstärkende Folie und zur Reduzierung der Streustrahlung eine Kassette mit stehendem Raster zu verwenden.
Der Zentralstrahl sollte die Mitte der Gliedmaße fingerbreit proximal des lateralen Kondylus der Tibia treffen und im rechten Winkel auf die Kassette einfallen.

Fig. 101 Positioning of stifle joint. Lateromedial.

In the standing — if necessary sedated — horse the cassette is held perpendicularly, placed against the medial aspect of the stifle joint and pushed proximally as far as possible between the leg and the abdominal wall.
High definition screens should be used to depict fine details, providing the capacity of the X-ray machin is sufficient. Otherwise, standard screens should be used. To reduce scattered radiation, a cassette with a stationary grid is necessary.
The central beam should strike the center of the limb a fingerwidth proximal to the lateral condyle of the tibia and fall at right angles to the cassette.

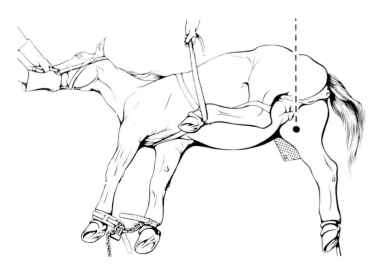

Abb. 102 Lagerung zur Aufnahme des Kniegelenks, liegend. Medio-lateral.

Eine bessere Aufnahme ist am liegenden Pferd bei medio-lateralem Strahlengang zu erzielen, weil eine feinzeichnende Folie, eine Bucky-Blende verwendet und eine längere Belichtungszeit (Narkose) in Kauf genommen werden können.
Bei der Lagerung ist darauf zu achten, daß die untenliegende Gliedmaße, gegebenenfalls unter leichtem Verkanten des Rumpfes, so weit vorgezogen wird, bis das distale Femurdrittel ohne Überlagerung durch das Abdomen dargestellt werden kann.
Der Zentralstrahl sollte die Mitte der Gliedmaße fingerbreit proximal des medialen Kondylus der Tibia treffen und im rechten Winkel auf die Kassette einfallen.

Fig. 102 Positioning of stifle joint, recumbent. Mediolateral.

With the beam directed mediolaterally a better radiograph can be obtained in lateral recumbency because high definition screens and a Bucky diaphragm can be used, and the exposure time can be extended (anesthesia).
In positioning, care must be taken to place the lower limb in such a manner that the distal third of the femur is free from overlaying by the abdomen — if necessary, the trunk may be rotated slightly.
The central beam should strike the center of the limb a fingerwidth proximal to the medial condyle of the tibia and fall at right angles to the cassette.

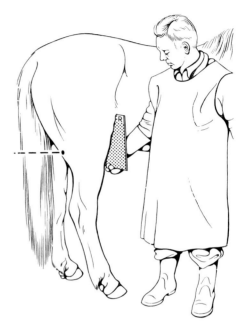

Abb. 103 Lagerung zur Aufnahme des Kniegelenks. Kaudo-kranial.

Die dem Kniegelenk kranial angelegte Kassette ist kräftig nach proximal und medial vorzuschieben. Diese Manipulation ist nur bei ruhigen Pferden ohne Sedierung möglich.
Zur Reduzierung der Streustrahlung ist eine Kassette mit stehendem Raster notwendig.
Der Zentralstrahl sollte die Mitte der Gliedmaße fingerbreit proximal des medialen Kondylus der Tibia treffen und im rechten Winkel auf die Kassette einfallen.

Fig. 103 Positioning of stifle joint. Caudocranial.

The cassette, placed against the cranial aspect of the stifle joint, should be pushed firmly in a proximal and medial direction. This manipulation is only possible without sedation in calm horses.
To reduce scattered radiation, a cassette with a stationary grid should be used.
The central beam should strike the middle of the limb a fingerwidth proximal to the medial condyle of the tibia and fall at right angles to the cassette.

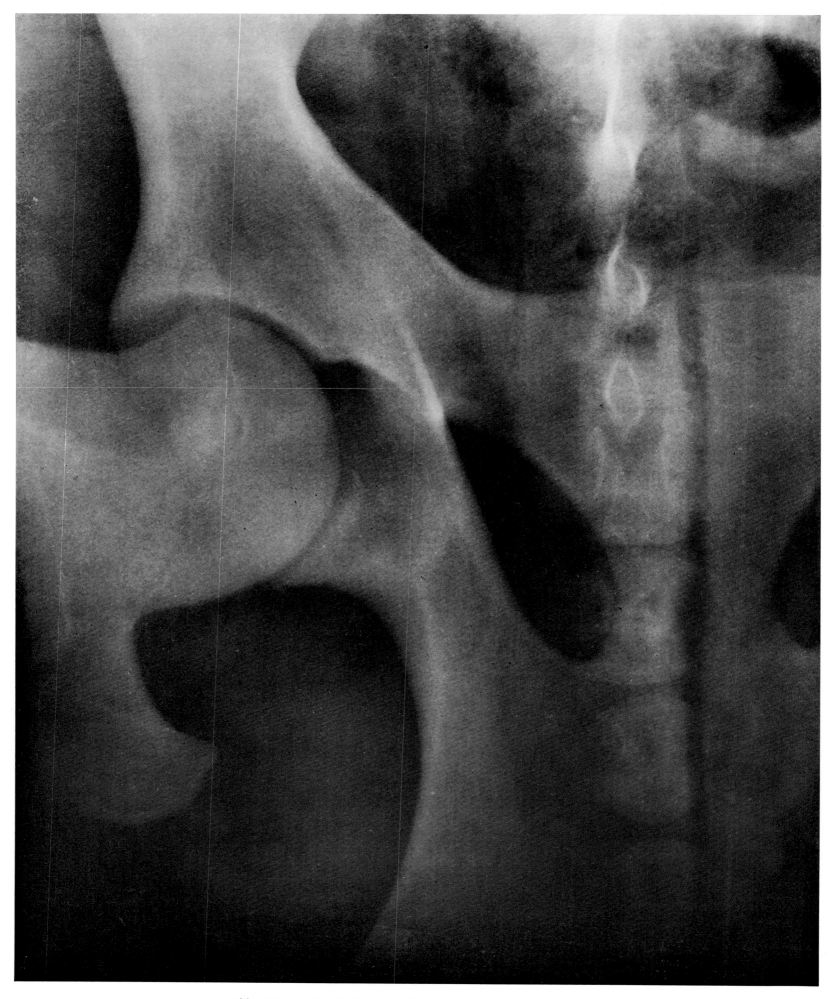

Abb. 104 Rechtes Hüftgelenk. Ventro-dorsal. Warmblut, 2 Jahre.
Bucky-Blende — Feinzeichnende Folie — FFA 100 cm — 85 kV — 400 mAs
Originalgröße (Ausschnitt aus 30 × 40 cm)
Lagerung Abb. 100

Fig. 104 Right hip joint. Ventrodorsal. Light horse, 2 years old.
Bucky diaphragm — High definition screens — FFD 100 cm — 85 kV — 400 mAs
Original size (section of 30 × 40 cm)
Positioning fig. 100

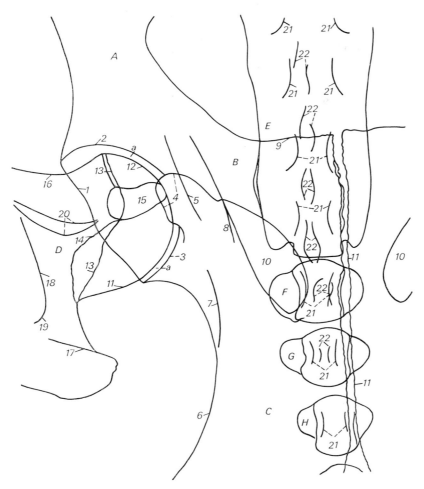

Abb. 105 Röntgenskizze zu Abb. 104 Fig. 105 X-ray sketch to fig. 104

A   Os ilium;
B   Os pubis;
C   Os ischii;
D   Os femoris;
E   Os sacrum;
F   1. Vertebra caudalis;
G   2. Vertebra caudalis;
H   3. Vertebra caudalis;

a   Articulatio coxae;

Am Becken — On the pelvis:

1   Acetabulum, dorsaler Rand — Acetabulum, dorsal border;
2, 3 Verschattungen, die sich aus der Konkavität des Acetabulums als kraniale (2) und kaudale (3) Begrenzung ergeben — Shadows formed by the concavity of the acetabulum as cranial (2) and caudal (3) borders;
4   Fossa et Incisura acetabuli;
5   Spina ischiadica;
6   Incisura ischiadica minor;
7   Verschattung, die sich aus der Konkavität an der lateralen Fläche des Corpus ossis ischii ergibt — Shadow formed by the concavity of the lateral surface of the body of ischium;
8   Corpus ossis ilium, orthograph getroffene Kompakta an der medialen Seitenfläche — Corpus ossis ilium, orthographically struck compacta of the medial surface;
9   Pecten ossis pubis et Eminentia iliopectinea;

10 Foramen obturatum;
11 Symphysis pelvina;

Am Os femoris — On the femur:

12 Caput ossis femoris,
13, 14 Kraniale (13) und kaudale (14) Begrenzung seiner Facies articularis — Cranial (13) and caudal (14) borders of its articular surface;
15 Fovea capitis;
16 Collum ossis femoris;
17 Trochanter major, Pars caudalis, kaudomedialer Rand — Trochanter major, pars caudalis, caudomedial border;
18 Trochanter major, Pars cranialis, orthograph getroffene Basis — Trochanter major, pars cranialis, orthographically struck base;
19 Incisura trochanterica, orthograph getroffene Basis — Incisura trochanterica, orthographically struck base;
20 Verschattung, die sich aus der Konkavität an der Basis des Trochanter minor ergibt — Shadow formed by the concavity of the base of the lesser trochanter;

Am Kreuzbein und an den Schwanzwirbeln — On the sacrum and caudal vertebrae:

21 Canalis vertebrae, seitliche Begrenzung — Canalis vertebrae, lateral border;
22 Verschattungen, die sich aus orthograph getroffenen Abschnitten der Processus spinosi ergeben — Shadows formed by the orthographically struck parts of the spinous processes.

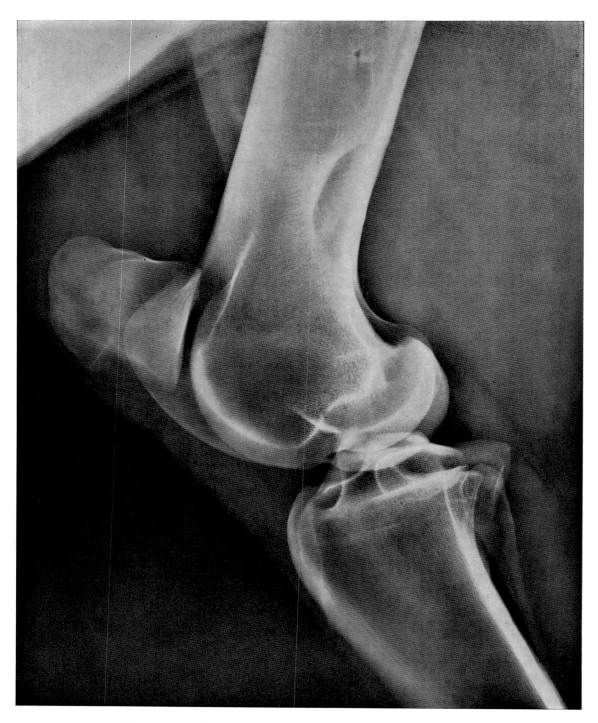

Abb. 106   Rechtes Kniegelenk. Medio-lateral. Warmblut, 3 Jahre.
Bucky-Blende — Feinzeichnende Folie — FFA 100 cm — 65 kV — 50 mAs
Verkleinerung von 30 × 40 cm
Lagerung Abb. 102

Fig. 106   Right stifle joint. Mediolateral. Light horse, 3 years old.
Bucky diaphragm — High definition screens — FFD 100 cm — 65 kV — 50 mAs
Diminution of 30 × 40 cm
Positioning fig. 102

A   Os femoris;
B   Patella;
C   Tibia;
D   Fibula;

a   Articulatio femoropatellaris;
b   Articulatio femorotibialis;

Am Os femoris — On the femur:

1—3   Trochlea ossis femoris:
1   Lateraler Rollkamm — Lateral ridge,
2   Medialer Rollkamm — Medial ridge,

3   Rollfurche — Groove of the trochlea;
4   Fossa extensoria;
5   Condylus lateralis;
6   Condylus medialis;
7   Fossa intercondylaris;
8   Facies poplitea;
9   Fossa supracondylaris;
10   Labium laterale, nach proximal in die Basis des Trochanter tertius übergehend — Labium laterale, changing proximally into the base of the trochanter tertius;
11   Labium mediale;
12   Foramen nutricium;

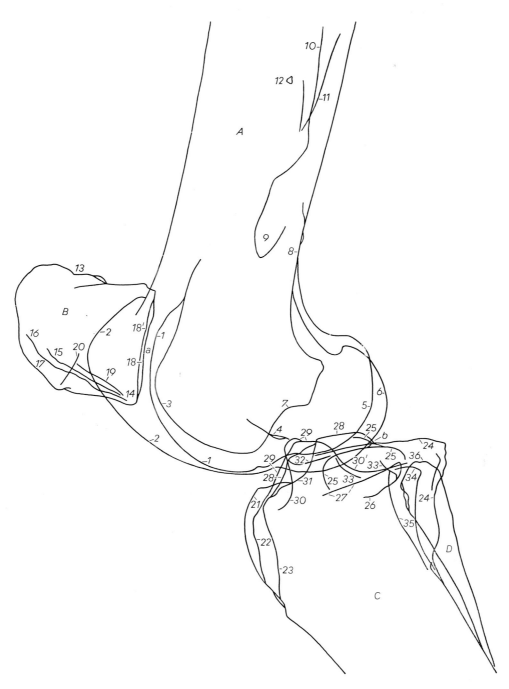

Abb. 107 Röntgenskizze zu Abb. 106   Fig. 107 X-ray sketch to fig. 106

An der Patella — On the patella:

13 Basis patellae;
14 Apex patellae;
15—17 Facies cranialis:
15 Lateraler Rand — Lateral border,
16 Dorsaler Rand — Dorsal border,
17 Medialer Rand — Medial border;
18 Facies articularis,
18' Führungskamm — Ridge;
19, 20 Kompaktaschatten, der sich aus der Wölbung der Facies articularis (19) sowie aus ihrer Konkavität (20) zum medialen Rollkamm hin ergibt — Compacta shadow formed by the curvature (19) and concavity (20) of the articular surface towards the medial ridge of the trochlea;

An der Tibia — On the tibia:

21, 22 Tuberositas tibiae:
21 Lateraler Abschnitt — Lateral part,
22 Medialer Abschnitt — Medial part;
23 Bandgrube zwischen 21 und 22 — Groove for ligamentous attachment between 21 and 22;
24 Condylus lateralis;

25 Verschattungen, die sich aus der Wölbung der Facies articularis des Condylus lateralis ergeben — Shadows formed by the curvature of the articular surface of the lateral condyle;
26 Condylus medialis;
27 Facies articularis;
28 Tuberculum intercondylare laterale;
29 Tuberculum intercondylare mediale;
30, 30' Kranialer bzw. kaudaler Rand der am Tuberculum intercondylare mediale aufsteigenden Gelenkfläche des Condylus medialis — Cranial and caudal borders of the articular surface of the medial condyle respectively continuing proximally along the medial intercondylar tubercle;
31, 32, 33 Verschattungen, die sich aus der Konkavität der Area intercondylaris cranialis lateralis (31), der Area intercondylaris centralis (32) und der Area intercondylaris caudalis (33) ergeben — Shadows formed by the concavity of the lateral cranial intercondylar area (31), the central intercondylar area (32) and the caudal intercondylar area (33);
34 Area intercondylaris caudalis, nasenförmige Verlängerung — Area intercondylaris caudalis, elongation;
35 Verschattung, die sich aus der Konkavität der Incisura poplitea ergibt — Shadow formed by the concavity of the popliteal incisure;
36 Caput fibulae.

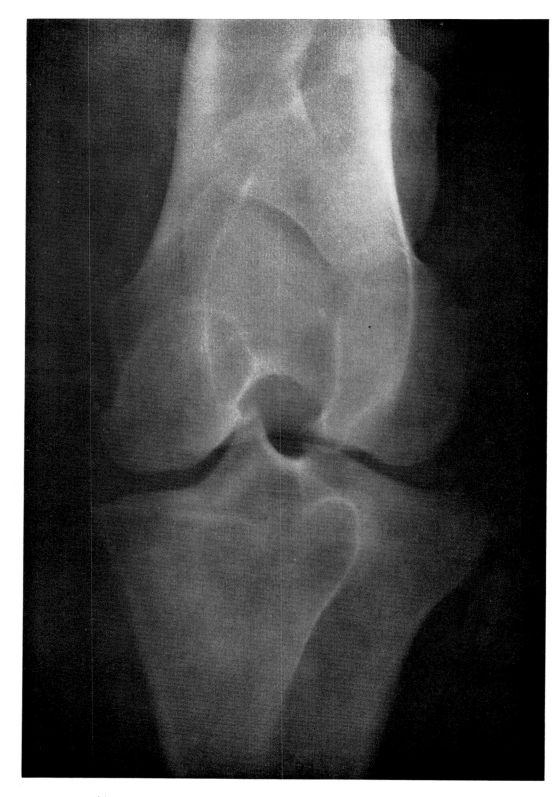

Abb. 108   Rechtes Kniegelenk. Kaudo-kranial. Warmblut, 16 Jahre.
Bucky-Blende — Feinzeichnende Folie — FFA 100 cm — 70 kV — 98 mAs
Verkleinerung von 24 × 30 cm
Lagerung Abb. 103

Fig. 108   Right stifle joint. Caudocranial. Light horse, 16 years old.
Bucky diaphragm — High definition screens — FFD 100 cm — 70 kV — 98 mAs
Diminution of 24 × 30 cm
Positioning fig. 103

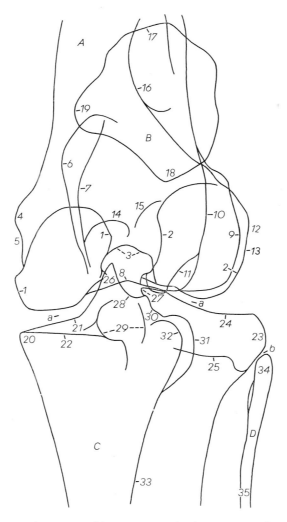

Abb. 109 Röntgenskizze zu Abb. 108   Fig. 109 X-ray sketch to fig. 108

A   Os femoris;
B   Patella;
C   Tibia;
D   Fibula;

a   Articulatio femorotibialis;
b   Articulatio tibiofibularis;

Am Os femoris — On the femur:
1   Condylus medialis;
2   Condylus lateralis;
3   Fossa intercondylaris;
4   Medialer Bandhöcker — Medial eminence for ligamentous attachment;
5   Mediale Bandgrube — Medial depression for ligamentous attachment;
6   Begrenzung des medialen Rollkamms — Border of the medial ridge of the trochlea;
7   Verschattung, die sich aus der Konkavität an der Basis des medialen Rollkamms ergibt — Shadow formed by the concavity at the base of the medial ridge of the trochlea;
8   Rollfurche — Groove between the ridges of the trochlea;
9   Begrenzung des lateralen Rollkamms — Border of the lateral ridge of the trochlea;
10   Verschattung, die sich aus der Konkavität an der Basis des lateralen Rollkamms ergibt — Shadow formed by the concavity at the base of the lateral ridge of the trochlea;
11   Verschattung, die sich aus der Konkavität der Fossa extensoria ergibt — Shadow formed by the concavity of the extensor fossa;
12   Lateraler Bandhöcker — Lateral eminence for ligamentous attachment;
13   Laterale Bandgrube — Lateral depression for ligamentous attachment;
14, 15   Insertionsstelle des Ligamentum cruciatum caudale (14) bzw. Ligamentum cruciatum craniale (15) — Insertions of the ligamentum cruciatum caudale (14) and ligamentum cruciatum craniale (15) respectively;
16   Fossa supracondylaris, mediale Begrenzung — Fossa supracondylaris, medial border;

An der Patella — On the patella:
17   Basis patellae;
18   Apex patellae;
19   Processus cartilagineus;

An der Tibia — On the tibia:
20   Condylus medialis,
21, 22   Facies articularis:
21   Proximale Begrenzung — Proximal border,
22   Kaudale Begrenzung — Caudal border;
23   Condylus lateralis,
24, 25   Facies articularis:
24   Proximale Begrenzung — Proximal border,
25   Kaudale Begrenzung (abschnittsweise dargestellt) — Caudal border (partly shown);
26, 27   Eminentia intercondylaris:
26   Tuberculum intercondylare mediale,
27   Tuberculum intercondylare laterale;
28   Area intercondylaris centralis;
29   Area intercondylaris caudalis, Begrenzung — Area intercondylaris caudalis, border;
30   Area intercondylaris cranialis lateralis, kraniomediale Begrenzung — Area intercondylaris cranialis lateralis, craniomedial border;
31   Tuberositas tibiae;
32   Verschattung, die sich aus der Wölbung des Sulcus extensorius ergibt — Shadow formed by the curvature of the extensor groove;
33   Margo cranialis;

An der Fibula — On the fibula:
34   Caput fibulae;
35   Corpus fibulae.

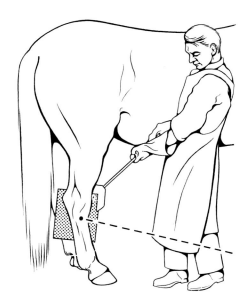

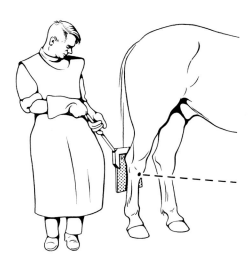

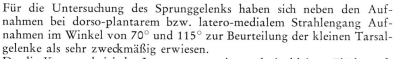

Abb. 110   Lagerung zur Aufnahme des Tarsalgelenks. Latero-medial.

Fig. 110   Positioning of hock joint. Lateromedial.

Abb. 111   Lagerung zur Aufnahme des Tarsalgelenks. Dorso-plantar.

Fig. 111   Positioning of hock joint. Dorsoplantar.

Für die Untersuchung des Sprunggelenks haben sich neben den Aufnahmen bei dorso-plantarem bzw. latero-medialem Strahlengang Aufnahmen im Winkel von 70° und 115° zur Beurteilung der kleinen Tarsalgelenke als sehr zweckmäßig erwiesen.

Da die Kassette bei jeder Lagerung nur einer relativ kleinen Fläche aufliegt, sind Verkantungen leicht möglich. Um diesen vorzubeugen, sollte man, falls ein Lichtvisier vorhanden ist, auf der Kassette Strichmarkierungen anbringen und auf diese im vorgesehenen Abstand vor der Kassettenlagerung ausblenden.

Zur Reduzierung der Streustrahlung ist eine Kassette mit stehendem Raster erforderlich.

Der Zentralstrahl sollte fingerbreit distal der Rollkämme des Talus die Mitte der Gliedmaße von dorsal (Abb. 111), von lateral im Winkel von 90° (Abb. 110), von lateral im Winkel von 70° (Abb. 112) und von lateral im Winkel von 115° (Abb. 113) treffen und jeweils im rechten Winkel auf die Kassette einfallen.

In addition to the dorsoplantar and lateromedial directions of the beam in radiography of the hock joint, radiographs taken at angles of 70° and 115° proved to be most satisfactory in evaluating the small tarsal joints.

Since, in any position, the cassette contacts only relatively small surface area, tilting is easily possible. If a multileaf collimator with light beam diaphragm is available, tilting can be eliminated before placing by adjusting the shutter according to the desired distance and area to be examined.

A stationary grid will be necessary to reduce scattered radiation.

The central beam should strike the center of the limb on the dorsal aspect, a fingerwidth distal to the troplea of the talus (fig. 111), from the lateral aspect at a right angle (fig. 110), an angle of 70° (fig. 112) and an angle of 115° (fig. 113). In each case the beam should fall at right angles to the cassette.

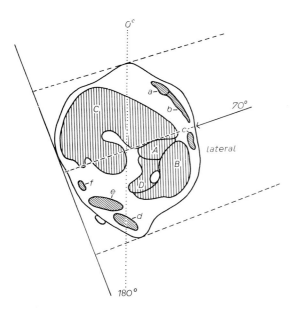

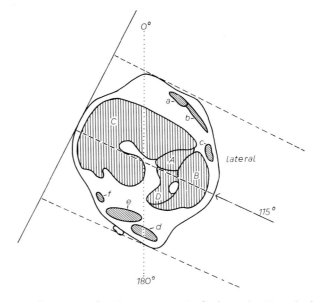

Abb. 112 Lagerung der Kassette zur Aufnahme des Tarsalgelenks.
Kraniolateral-kaudomedial (70°).

Fig. 112 Positioning of the cassette for the hock joint.
Craniolateral-caudomedial (70°).

Abb. 113 Lagerung der Kassette zur Aufnahme des Tarsalgelenks.
Kaudolateral-kraniomedial (115°).

Fig. 113 Positioning of the cassette for the hock joint.
Caudolateral-craniomedial (115°).

Horizontalschnitt durch das rechte Tarsalgelenk eines Pferdes in Höhe
des Os tarsi centrale.

Horizontal section through the right hock joint of the horse at the level
of the central tarsal bone.

A Talus;
B Calcaneus;
C Os tarsi centrale;
D Os tarsale IV;

a Sehne des M. extensor digitalis longus — Tendon of m. extensor digitalis longus;
b M. extensor digitalis brevis;
c Sehne des M. extensor digitalis lateralis — Tendon of m. extensor digitalis lateralis;
d Sehne des M. flexor digitalis superficialis — Tendon of m. flexor digitalis superficialis;
e Sehnen der Mm. flexor hallucis longus et tibialis caudalis — Tendons of m. flexor hallucis longus and m. tibialis caudalis;
f Sehne des M. flexor digitalis longus — Tendon of m. flexor digitalis longus.

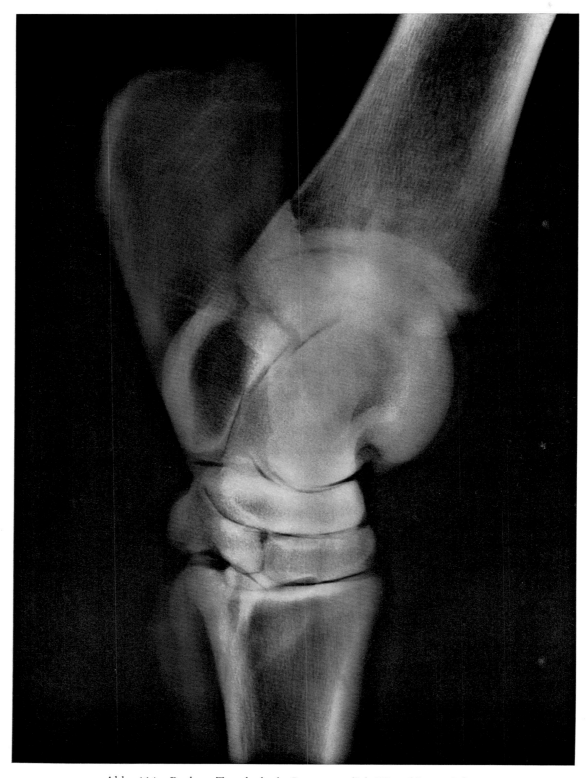

Abb. 114   Rechtes Tarsalgelenk. Latero-medial. Warmblut, 9 Jahre.
Stehendes Raster — Feinzeichnnende Folie — FFA 100 cm — 65 kV — 40 mAs
Verkleinerung von 24 × 30 cm
Lagerung Abb. 110

Fig. 114   Right hock joint. Lateromedial. Light horse, 9 years old.
Stationary grid — High definition screens — FFD 100 cm — 65 kV — 40 mAs
Diminution of 24 × 30 cm
Positioning fig. 110

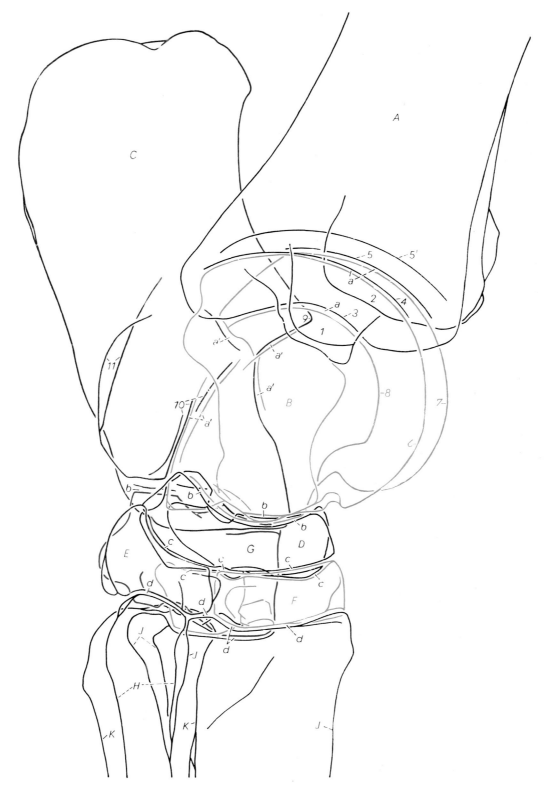

Abb. 115** Röntgenskizze zu Abb. 114   Fig. 115** X-ray sketch to fig. 114

A   Tibia;
B   Talus;
C   Calcaneus;
D   Os tarsi centrale;
E   Os tarsale I et II;
F   Os tarsale III;
G   Os tarsale IV;
H   Os metatarsale II;
J   Os metatarsale III;
K   Os metatarsale IV;

a   Articulatio tarsocruralis;
a′   Gelenkspalte zwischen Talus und Calcaneus — Joint space between talus and calcaneus;
b   Articulationes talocalcaneocentralis et calcaneoquartalis;
c   Articulatio centrodistalis;
d   Articulationes tarsometatarseae;

1   Malleolus medialis;
2   Malleolus lateralis;

3–5′ Cochlea tibiae:
3   Sagittalkamm — Sagittal ridge,
4   Mediale Rollfurche — Medial groove,
5   Laterale Rollfurche — Lateral groove,
5′   Verschattung, die sich aus den Kompaktaverstärkungen der beiden Rollfurchen ergibt — Shadow formed by the increased compacta of both grooves;
6–8 Trochlea tali:
6   Medialer Rollkamm — Medial ridge,
7   Lateraler Rollkamm — Lateral ridge,
8   Verschattung, die sich aus der Konkavität am Grund Der Rollfurche ergibt — Shadow formed by the concavity at the base of the groove;
9   Processus coracoideus;
10   Verschattungen, die sich aus Kompaktaverstärkungen am Sustentaculum tali ergeben — Shadows formed by the increased compacta of the sustentaculum tali;
11   Begrenzungen der Sehnenrinne der Mm. flexor hallucis longus et tibialis caudalis am Sustentaculum tali — Borders of the groove for the tendon of m. flexor hallucis longus and m. tibialis caudalis on the sustentaculum tali.

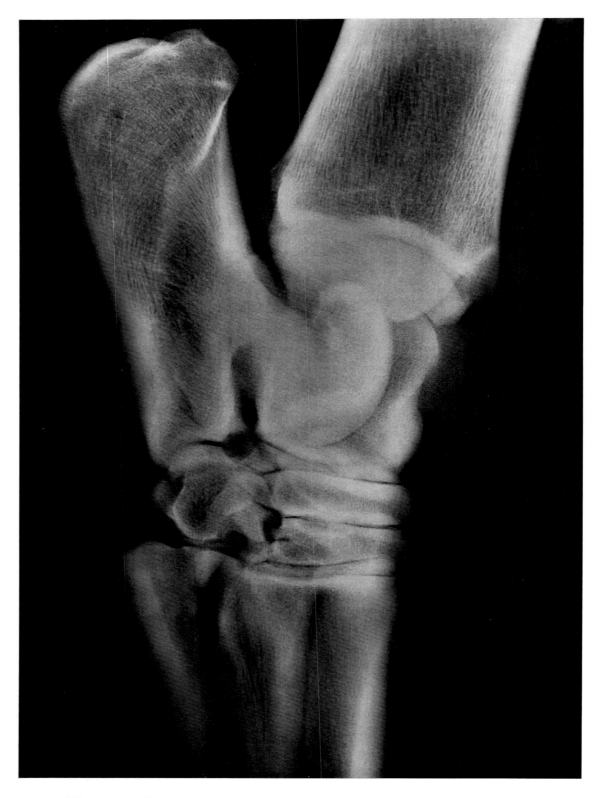

Abb. 116   Rechtes Tarsalgelenk. Kraniolateral-kaudomedial (70°). Warmblut, 9 Jahre.
Stehendes Raster — Feinzeichnende Folie — FFA 100 cm — 65 kV — 40 mAs
Verkleinerung von 24 × 30 cm
Lagerung Abb. 112

Fig. 116   Right hock joint. Craniolateral-caudomedial (70°). Light horse, 9 years old.
Stationary grid — High definition screens — FFD 100 cm — 65 kV — 40 mAs
Diminution of 24 × 30 cm
Positioning fig. 112

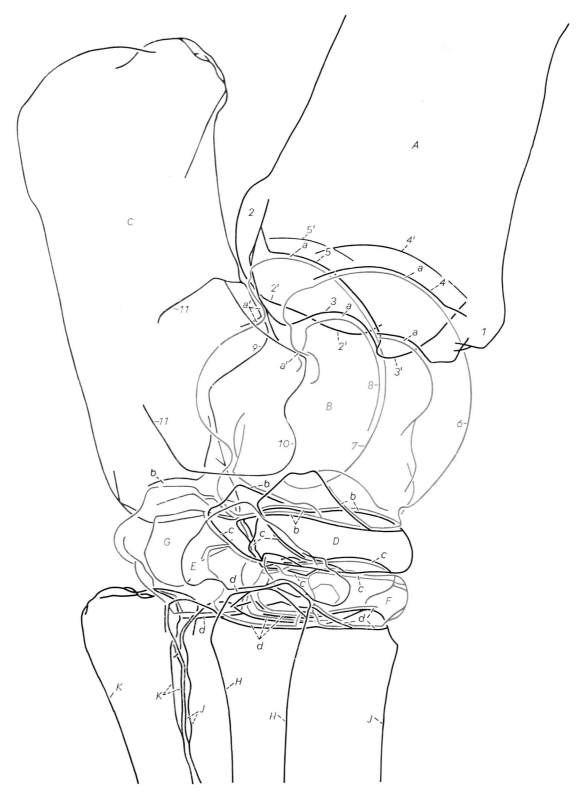

Abb. 117** Röntgenskizze zu Abb. 116   Fig. 117** X-ray sketch to fig. 116

A Tibia;
B Talus;
C Calcaneus;
D Os tarsi centrale;
E Os tarsale I et II;
F Os tarsale III;
G Os tarsale IV;
H Os metatarsale II;
J Os metatarsale III;
K Os metatarsale IV;

a Articulatio tarsocruralis;
a′ Gelenkspalte zwischen Talus und Calcaneus — Joint space between talus and calcaneus;
b Articulationes talocalcaneocentralis et calcaneoquartalis;
c Articulatio centrodistalis;
d Articulationes tarsometatarseae;

1 Malleolus medialis;
2 Malleolus lateralis;
2′—5′ Cochlea tibiae:
2′ Laterale Begrenzung — Lateral border,

3 Sagittalkamm — Sagittal ridge,
3′ Dorsale Kante — Dorsal edge,
4 Mediale Rollfurche — Medial groove,
4′ Verschattung, die sich aus der Kompaktaverstärkung der medialen Rollfurche ergibt — Shadow formed by the increased compacta of the medial groove,
5 Laterale Rollfurche — Lateral groove,
5′ Verschattung, die sich aus der Kompaktaverstärkung der lateralen Rollfurche ergibt — Shadow formed by the increased compacta of the lateral groove;
6—8 Trochlea tali:
6 Medialer Rollkamm — Medial ridge,
7 Lateraler Rollkamm — Lateral ridge,
8 Verschattung, die sich aus der Konkavität am Grund der Rollfurche ergibt — Shadow formed by the concavity at the base of the groove;
9 Processus coracoideus;
10 Sustentaculum tali;
11 Begrenzungen der Sehnenrinne der Mm. flexor hallucis longus et tibialis caudalis am Sustentaculum tali — Borders of the groove for the tendon of m. flexor hallucis longus and m. tibialis caudalis on the sustentaculum tali.

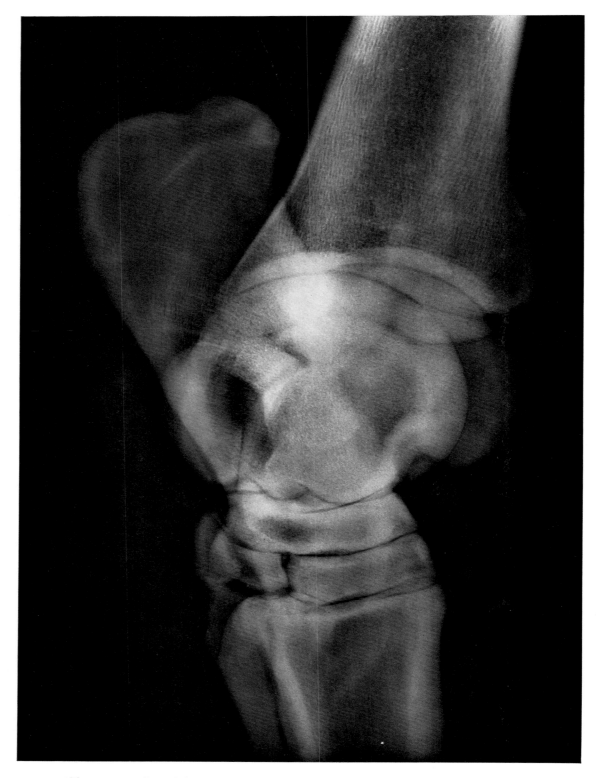

Abb. 118   Rechtes Tarsalgelenk. Kaudolateral-kraniomedial (115°). Warmblut, 9 Jahre.
Stehendes Raster — Feinzeichnende Folie — FFA 100 cm — 65 kV — 40 mAs
Verkleinerung von 24 × 30 cm
Lagerung Abb. 113

Fig. 118   Right hock joint. Caudolateral-craniomedial (115°). Light horse, 9 years old.
Stationary grid — High definition screens — FFD 100 cm — 65 kV — 40 mAs
Diminution of 24 × 30 cm
Positioning fig. 113

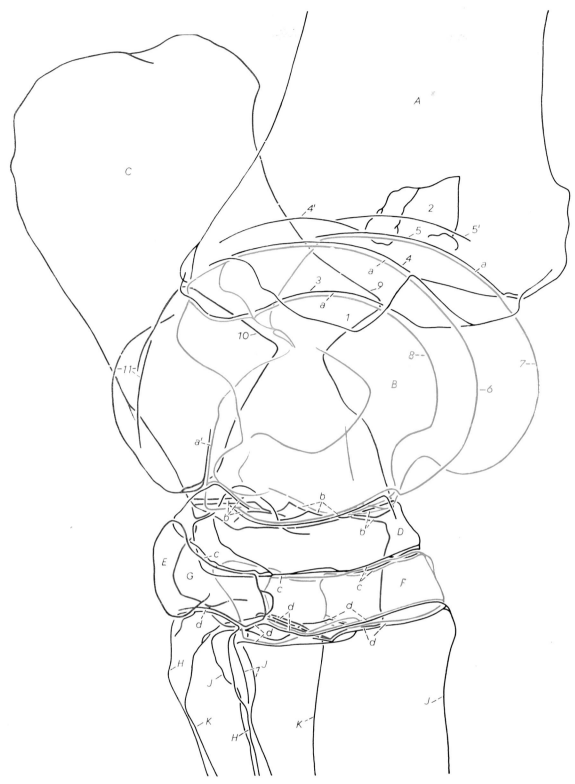

Abb. 119** Röntgenskizze zu Abb. 118   Fig. 119** X-ray sketch to fig. 118

A   Tibia;
B   Talus;
C   Calcaneus;
D   Os tarsi centrale;
E   Os tarsale I et II;
F   Os tarsale III;
G   Os tarsale IV;
H   Os metatarsale II;
J   Os metatarsale III;
K   Os metatarsale IV;

a   Articulatio tarsocruralis;
a'   Gelenkspalte zwischen Talus und Calcaneus — Joint space between talus and calcaneus;
b   Articulationes talocalcaneocentralis et calcaneoquartalis;
c   Articulatio centrodistalis;
d   Articulationes tarsometatarseae;

1   Malleolus medialis;
2   Sehnenrinne auf dem Malleolus lateralis — Groove for tendon on the lateral malleolus;

3—5'   Cochlea tibiae:
3   Sagittalkamm — Sagittal ridge,
4   Mediale Rollfurche — Medial groove,
4'   Verschattung, die sich aus der Kompaktaverstärkung der medialen Rollfurche ergibt — Shadow formed by the increased compacta of the medial groove,
5   Laterale Rollfurche — Lateral groove,
5'   Verschattung, die sich aus der Kompaktaverstärkung der lateralen Rollfurche ergibt — Shadow formed by the increased compacta of the lateral groove;
6—8   Trochlea tali:
6   Medialer Rollkamm — Medial ridge,
7   Lateraler Rollkamm — Lateral ridge,
8   Verschattung, die sich aus der Konkavität am Grund der Rollfurche ergibt — Shadow formed by the concavity at the base of the groove;
9   Processus coracoideus;
10   Sustentaculum tali;
11   Begrenzungen der Sehnenrinne der Mm. flexor hallucis longus et tibialis caudalis am Sustentaculum tali — Borders of the groove for the tendon of m. flexor hallucis longus and m. tibialis caudalis on the sustentaculum tali.

94

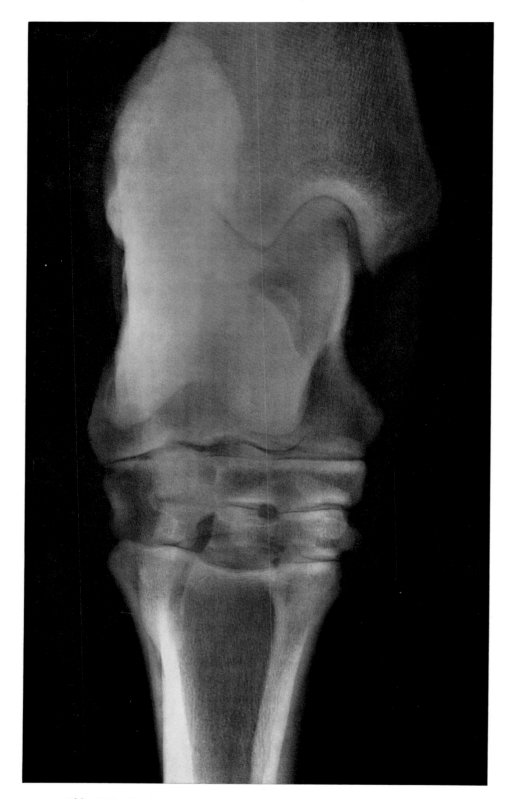

Abb. 120   Rechtes Tarsalgelenk. Dorso-plantar. Warmblut, 3 Jahre.
Stehendes Raster — Feinzeichnende Folie — FFA 100 cm — 65 kV — 90 mAs
Verkleinerung von 24 × 30 cm
Lagerung Abb. 111

Fig. 120   Right hock joint. Dorsoplantar. Light horse, 3 years old.
Stationary grid — High definition screens — FFD 100 cm — 65 kV — 90 mAs
Diminution of 24 × 30 cm
Positioning fig. 111

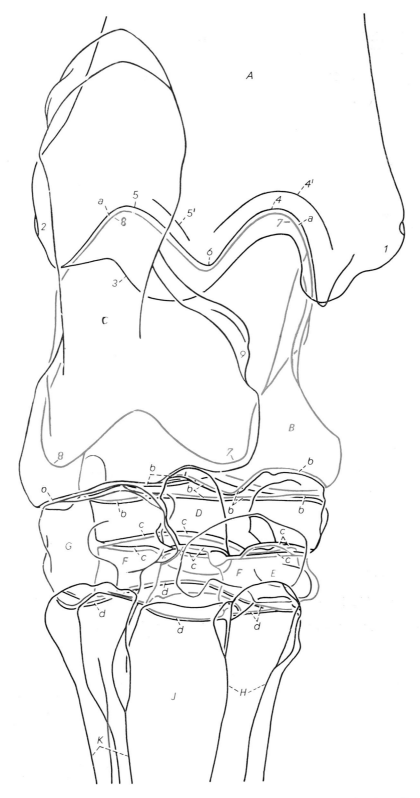

Abb. 121** Röntgenskizze zu Abb. 120   Fig. 121** X-ray sketch to fig. 120

A	Tibia;	1	Malleolus medialis;
B	Talus;	2	Malleolus lateralis;
C	Calcaneus;	3–6	Cochlea tibiae:
D	Os tarsi centrale;	3	Kraniale Begrenzung — Cranial border,
E	Os tarsale I et II;	4	Mediale Rollfurche — Medial groove,
F	Os tarsale III;	4′	Verschattung, die sich aus der Kompaktaverstärkung der medialen Rollfurche ergibt — Shadow formed by the increased compacta of the medial groove,
G	Os tarsale IV;	5	Laterale Rollfurche — Lateral groove,
H	Os metatarsale II;	5′	Verschattung, die sich aus der Kompaktaverstärkung der lateralen Rollfurche ergibt — Shadow formed by the increased compacta of the lateral groove,
J	Os metatarsale III;	6	Sagittalkamm — Sagittal ridge;
K	Os metatarsale IV;	7, 8	Trochlea tali:
		7	Medialer Rollkamm — Medial ridge,
a	Articulatio tarsocruralis;	8	Lateraler Rollkamm — Lateral ridge;
b	Articulationes talocalcaneocentralis et calcaneoquartalis;	9	Sustentaculum tali.
c	Articulatio centrodistalis;		
d	Articulationes tarsometatarseae;		

Lagerung der Kassette zur Aufnahme der Griffelbeine.

Zur Aufnahme der Griffelbeine ergeben sich die in den Abbildungen 122 und 123 dargestellten Möglichkeiten zur Lagerung der Kassette und die Einstellungen des Strahlengangs.

Der Zentralstrahl sollte das Griffelbein im mittleren Drittel treffen und im rechten Winkel auf die Kassette einfallen.

Positioning of the cassette for the splint bones.

In radiographing the splint bones, various possibilities of placing the cassette and focusing the beam are shown in figs. 122 and 123.

The central beam should strike the splint bone in the middle third and fall at right angles to the cassette.

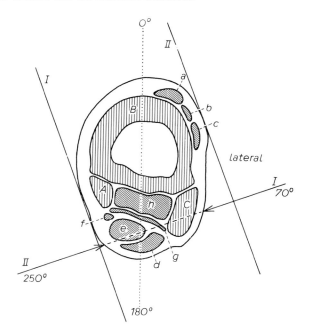

Abb. 122 Lagerung der Kassette zur Darstellung des lateralen Griffelbeins der rechten Beckengliedmaße.

Fig. 122 Positioning of the cassette for the lateral splint bone of the right pelvic limb.

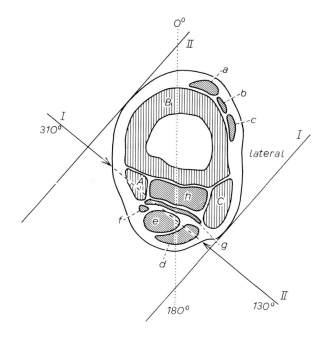

Abb. 123 Lagerung der Kassette zur Darstellung des medialen Griffelbeins der rechten Beckengliedmaße.

Fig. 123 Positioning of the cassette for the medial splint bone of the right pelvic limb.

A   Os metatarsale II;
B   Os metatarsale III;
C   Os metatarsale IV;

a   Sehne des M. extensor digitalis longus — Tendon of m. extensor digitalis longus;
b   Sehne des M. extensor digitalis brevis — Tendon of m. extensor digitalis brevis;
c   Sehne des M. extensor digitalis lateralis — Tendon of m. extensor digitalis lateralis;

d   Sehne des M. flexor digitalis superficialis — Tendon of m. flexor digitalis superficialis;
e   Sehnen der Mm. flexor hallucis longus et tibialis caudalis — Tendons of m. flexor hallucis longus and m. tibialis caudalis;
f   Sehne des M. flexor digitalis longus — Tendon of m. flexor digitalis longus;
g   Unterstützungsschenkel, Ligamentum accessorium — Tarsal check ligament, accessory ligament;
h   M. interosseus medius.

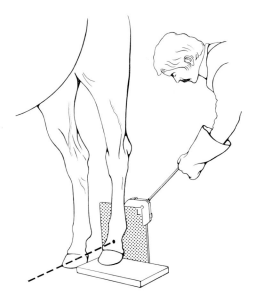

Abb. 124 Lagerung zur Aufnahme der Zehe. Dorso-plantar.

Zur Aufnahme des Fesselgelenks wird die Kassette senkrecht hinter dem Fesselkopf gelagert.

Der Zentralstrahl sollte die Mitte der Gliedmaßenvorderfläche in Höhe der distalen Gleichbeinkanten treffen und im rechten Winkel auf die Kassette einfallen.

Zur Aufnahme von Fessel- und Kronbein und zur Aufnahme des Krongelenks wird die Kassette dem Fesselkopf und dem Ballen angelegt.

Der Zentralstrahl sollte — abhängig von der Fragestellung — das Fesselbein in der Medianebene in halber Höhe bzw. das Krongelenk in der Mitte treffen und im rechten Winkel auf die Kassette einfallen.

Um den distalen Zehenbereich bei horizontalem Strahlengang aufnehmen zu können, ist die zu untersuchende Gliedmaße auf einen 5 cm starken Holzklotz so zu stellen, daß sich die Ballen über der Kante des Holzklotzes befinden. Wenn die aufzunehmende Gliedmaße wegen der Höherstellung nicht ausreichend belastet wird, empfiehlt es sich, die Schultergliedmaße derselben Seite wie zum Beschlag hochheben zu lassen.

Zur Zehenübersichtsaufnahme wird die Kassette dem Fesselkopf und dem Ballen angelegt.

Der Zentralstrahl sollte das Krongelenk in der Medianebene treffen und im rechten Winkel auf die Kassette einfallen.

Fig. 124 Positioning of digit. Dorsoplantar.

In radiographing the fetlock joint, the cassette should be placed perpendicularly behind the joint.

The central beam should strike the center of the dorsal surface of the digit on a level of the distal border of the sesamoid bone and fall at right angles to the cassette.

In radiographing the proximal and middle phalanges as well as the pastern joint, the cassette should be placed against the fetlock joint and the bulbs of the hoof.

Depending on the case in question, the central beam should strike the axis of the proximal phalanx at the middle of its length and the center of the pastern joint respectively and fall at right angles to the cassette.

In radiographing the distal digital region with a horizontal beam, it is necessary to place the extremity upon a wooden block approximately 5 cm thick. The bulbs of the hoof should be placed upon the edge of the block. When the leg to be examined does not bear sufficient weight, one hoof of the thoracic limb of the same side should be lifted and held up.

In routine radiography of the digit the cassette should be placed against the fetlock joint and the bulbs of the hoof.

The central beam should strike the center of the pastern joint and fall at right angles to the cassette.

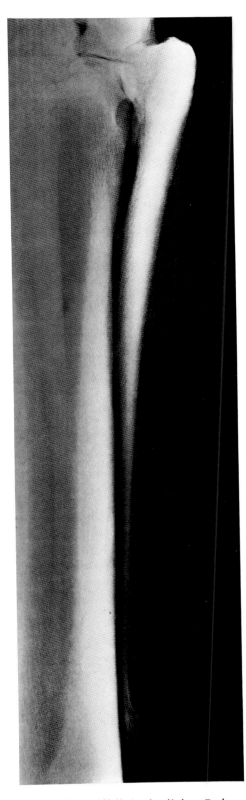

Abb. 125   Laterales Griffelbein der linken Beckengliedmaße.
Warmblut, 11 Jahre.
Feinzeichnende Folie — FFA 100 cm — 48 kV — 10 mAs
Verkleinerung von 24 × 30 cm
Lagerung Abb. 122

Fig. 125   Lateral splint bone of left pelvic limb.
Light horse, 11 years old.
High definition screens — FFD 100 cm — 48 kV — 10 mAs
Diminution of 24 × 30 cm
Positioning fig. 122

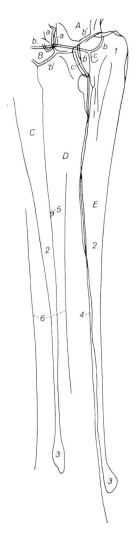

Abb. 126   Röntgenskizze zu Abb. 125
Fig. 126   X-ray sketch to fig. 125

A   Os tarsale III;
B   Os tarsale IV;
C   Os metatarsale II;
D   Os metatarsale III;
E   Os metatarsale IV;

a   Articulationes intertarseae;
b, b'   Articulationes tarsometatarseae:
b   Plantare Abschnitte — Plantar parts,
b'   Zentrale Abschnitte — Central parts;
c   Articulationes intermetatarseae;

Am Os metatarsale IV — On the 4th metatarsal bone:

1   Basis;
2   Corpus;
3   Caput;
4   Spalte zwischen Os metatarsale III und Os metatarsale IV zum Durchtritt des Ramus perforans distalis aus der A. metatarsea dorsalis III — Space between the 3rd and 4th metatarsal bones for the ramus perforans distalis of the a. metatarsea dorsalis III;

Am Os metatarsale III — On the 3rd metatarsal bone:

5   Foramen nutricium;
6   Cavum medullare.

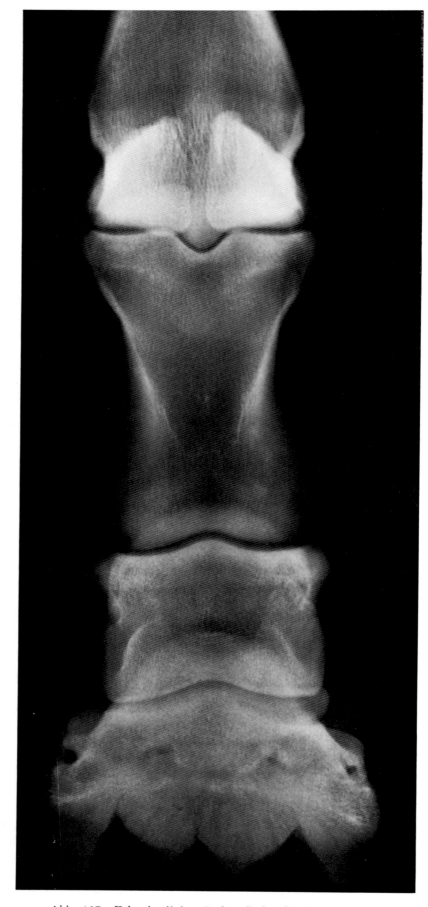

Abb. 127 Zehe der linken Beckengliedmaße. Dorso-plantar.
Traber, 5 Jahre.
Feinzeichnende Folie — FFA 100 cm — 58 kV — 20 mAs
Originalgröße
Lagerung Abb. 124

Fig. 127 Digit of left pelvic limb. Dorsoplantar.
Trotter, 5 years old.
High definition screens — FFD 100 cm — 58 kV — 20 mAs
Original size
Positioning fig. 124

A Os metatarsale III;
B Laterales Os sesamoideum proximale — Lateral proximal sesamoid bone;
C Mediales Os sesamoideum proximale — Medial proximal sesamoid bone;
D Phalanx proximalis;
E Phalanx media;
F Os sesamoideum distale;
G Phalanx distalis;
H Sporn, Calcar metatarseum — Ergot;

a Articulatio metatarsophalangea;
b Articulatio interphalangea proximalis;
c Articulatio interphalangea distalis;

Am Os metatarsale III — On the 3rd metatarsal bone:

1 Trochlea metatarsi, Sagittalkamm — Trochlea metatarsi, sagittal ridge;
2, 3 Facies articularis:
2 Plantare Begrenzung — Plantar limit,
3 Dorsale Begrenzung — Dorsal limit;
4 Bandhöcker — Eminence for ligamentous attachment;
5 Bandgrube — Depression for ligamentous attachment;

An den Ossa sesamoidea proximalia — On the proximal sesamoid bones:

6 Proximaler Randwulst — Proximal marginal thickening;
7 Facies articularis, laterale bzw. distale Begrenzung — Facies articularis, lateral and distal limits respectively;

An der Phalanx proximalis — On the proximal phalanx:

8, 9, 10 Basis et Fovea articularis:
8 Plantarer Rand — Plantar border,
9 Dorsaler Rand — Dorsal border,
10 Verschattung, die sich aus der Konkavität der Fovea articularis ergibt — Shadow formed by the concavity of the articular surface;
11 Bandhöcker — Eminence for ligamentous attachment;
12 Foramina nutricia;
13 Fesselbeinleisten — Ridges on the plantar surface;
14 Bandhöcker — Eminence for ligamentous attachment;
15 Bandgrube — Depression for ligamentous attachment;
16 Caput;
17, 18 Facies articularis:
17 Plantarer Rand — Plantar border,
18 Dorsaler Rand — Dorsal border;

An der Phalanx media — On the middle phalanx:

19—22 Basis et Fovea articularis:
19 Plantarer Rand — Plantar border,
20 Verschattung, die sich aus der Konkavität der Fovea articularis ergibt — Shadow formed by the concavity of the articular surface,
21 Dorsaler Rand — Dorsal border,
22 Kronbeinlehne — Transverse prominence for attachment of scutum medium;
23 Bandhöcker — Eminence for ligamentous attachment;
24 Verschattung, die sich aus der proximodorsalen Bandgrube ergibt — Shadow formed by the proximodorsal depression for ligamentous attachment;
25 Verschattung, die sich aus der distodorsalen Bandgrube ergibt — Shadow formed by the distodorsal depression for ligamentous attachment;
26 Caput;
27 Facies articularis, plantarer Rand, abschnittsweise dargestellt — Facies articularis, plantar border, only partly shown;

Am Os sesamoideum distale — On the distal sesamoid bone:

28 Margo proximalis;
29 Margo distalis;

An der Phalanx distalis — On the distal phalanx:

30 Facies articularis;
31 Processus extensorius;
32 Margo coronalis;
33, 34 Proximaler und distaler Ast des Processus plantaris medialis bzw. lateralis — Proximal and distal parts of the medial and lateral plantar processes respectively;

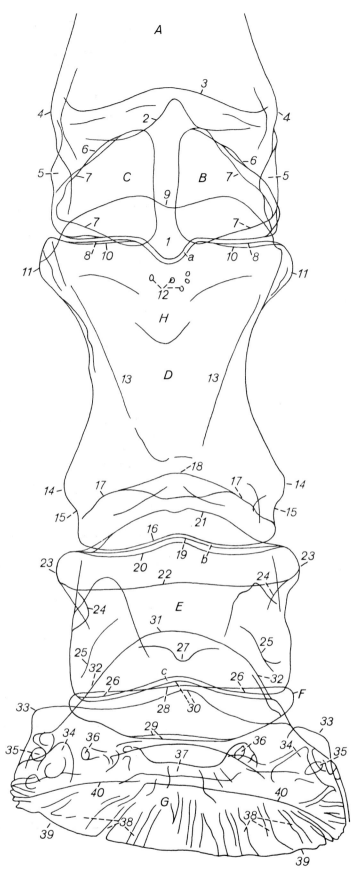

Abb. 128 Röntgenskizze zu Abb. 127

Fig. 128 X-ray sketch to fig. 127

35 Foramen processus plantaris;
36 Foramen soleare mediale bzw. Foramen soleare laterale — Medial and lateral solea foramina respectively;
37 Canalis solearis;
38 Gefäßkanäle — Vascular canals;
39 Margo solearis;
40 Facies solearis, orthograph getroffen — Facies solearis, orthographically struck.

Bibliographie Bibliography

ALKSNIS, A. (1938): Röntgenanatomische Studien über normale Gelenke beim Pferd, beim Hund und bei der Katze. Acta Univ. Latv. 2, 1

CAMPBELL, J. R., & R. LEE (1972): Radiological techniques in the diagnosis of navicular disease. Equine Vet. J. 4, 135

CARLSON, W. D. (1961): Veterinary radiology. Lea and Febiger, Philadelphia

COOK, W. R. (1973): The auditary tube diverticulum (guttural pouch) in the horse: its radiographic examination. J. Am. vet. Radiol. Soc. 14, 51

DOUGLAS, S. W., & H. D. WILLIAMSON (1963): Principles of veterinary radiography. Baillière, Tindall and Cox, London

ENGELHARDT, E. (1963): Röntgenanatomische Untersuchungen am Carpus des Pferdes. Hannover, Diss. med. vet.

GRATZL, E. (1944): Die klinische Diagnostik der katarrhalischen-entzündlichen Erkrankungen der oberen Luftwege des Pferdes mit besonderer Berücksichtigung der endoskopischen und röntgenologischen Untersuchungsmethoden. Z. Veterinärk. 56, 127

HABEL, R. E., R. B. BARRETT, C. D. DIESEM & W. J. ROENIGK (1963): Nomenclature for radiologic anatomy. J. Am. vet. med. Ass. 142, 38

HABERMANN, U. (1963): Zur röntgenologischen Darstellung der maxillaren Backenzähne des Pferdes. Hannover, Diss. med. vet.

HABERMEHL, K.-H. (1975): Altersbestimmung bei Haus -und Labortieren. 2. Aufl. Parey, Berlin — Hamburg

HARTUNG, K., W. CLAUS & H. KELLER (1968): Zum Strahlenschutz bei Röntgenaufnahmen in der Pferdepraxis (Personendosismessungen). Berl. Münch. tierärztl. Wschr. 81, 41

HEINZE, C. D., & R. E. LEWIS (1971): Radiographic examination of the equine pelvis: technique. J. Am. vet. med. Ass. 159, 1387

ILIJAŠ, B., F. SANCOVIĆ & K. BINEV (1968): A contribution to the X-ray diagnosis of pelvico-femoral bone lesions in large domestic animals. Zbl. Vet. Med. A 15, 322

JAHN, W. (1966): Die röntgenologisch nachweisbaren Veränderungen im Bereich der maxillaren Backenzähne des Pferdes in den verschiedenen Altersstufen. Hannover, Diss. med. vet.

JEFFCOTT, B. B. (1975): The diagnosis of the horse's back. Equine Vet. J. 7, 69

KÄNGSTRÖM, L. E. (1970): A simple technique for radiographic examination of the equine pelvis, hip joint and proximal femur. Proc. 2nd Int. Conf. Vet. Radiol., Stockholm. In: Acta radiol. Suppl. 319, 79 (1972)

KOVÁCS, G. H. (1954): Röntgenanatomie der vorderen Fußwurzelknochen des Pferdes. Acta vet. Acad. Scient. Hung. 4, 147

KOVÁCS, G. H. (1963): The equine tarsus. Akad. Kiadó, Budapest

KOVÁCS, G. H., L. GLOSZ & M. GERTNER (1964): Die Röntgenanatomie der Hirnschädelknochen des Pferdes. Acta vet. Acad. Scient. Hung. 14, 309

MEYER, B. (1964): Röntgen-anatomische Untersuchungen am Luftsack des Pferdes. Hannover, Diss. med. vet.

MORGAN, J. P. (1965): Radiographic study of the distal ulna of the horse. J. Am. vet. Radiol. Soc. 6, 78

MÜLLER, G. (1940): Röntgenatlas des Pferdes. Thieme, Leipzig

NICKEL, R., A. SCHUMMER & E. SEIFERLE (1975): Lehrbuch der Anatomie der Haustiere. II. Bd. Eingeweide. 3. Aufl. Parey, Berlin — Hamburg

NICKEL, R., A. SCHUMMER & E. SEIFERLE (1976): Lehrbuch der Anatomie der Haustiere. III. Bd. Kreislaufsystem, Haut und Hautorgane. Parey, Berlin — Hamburg

NICKEL, R., A. SCHUMMER & E. SEIFERLE (1977): Lehrbuch der Anatomie der Haustiere, I. Bd. Bewegungsapparat. 4. Aufl. Parey, Berlin — Hamburg

NOMINA ANATOMICA VETERINARIA (1973): Publ. by the Int. Committee on Vet. Anat. Nomenclature of the World Ass. of Vet. Anat., 2nd ed., Wien

OXSPRING, G. E. (1936): The radiology of navicular disease, with observations on its pathology. Vet. Rec. 15, 1443

PÖRSCHMANN, F. (1966): Zur röntgenologischen Darstellung der mandibularen Backenzähne des Pferdes unter Berücksichtigung verschiedener Altersstufen bis zum 3. Lebensjahr. Hannover, Diss. med. vet.

REID, F. R. (1965): Radiographic film. Identification and positioning. Proc. 11th A. Conv. Am. Ass. Equine Pract., 167

RYAN, G. D., & H. J. DEIGL (1969): Safety in large animal radiography. J. Am. vet. med. Ass. 155, 898

SASCHEK, M. (1964): Röntgen-anatomische Studie zum Spat des Pferdes. Hannover, Diss. med. vet.

SCHEBITZ, H. (1965): Zur Hemiplegia laryngis (Kehlkopfpfeifen) beim Pferd — Untersuchung und Operationsergebnis. Dtsch. tierärztl. Wschr. 72, 548

SCHEBITZ, H., & E. ENGELHARDT (1963): Zur Röntgenuntersuchung des Karpalgelenks vom Pferd. Tierärztl. Umschau 18, 416

SCHEBITZ, H., & W. WEBER (1963): Zur Röntgenuntersuchung des Gesichtsschädels vom Pferd. Dtsch. tierärztl. Wschr. 70, 450

SCHEBITZ, H., & H. WILKENS (1965): Zur röntgenologischen Untersuchung des Schultergelenks beim Pferd. Tierärztl. Umschau 20, 486

SCHEBITZ, H., & H. WILKENS (1967): Zum Spat des Pferdes — Untersuchung und Therapie. Berl. Münch. tierärztl. Wschr. 80, 385

SCHÖNHERR, P. (1958): Die Darstellung der Zähne des Pferdes im Röntgenbild. Leipzig, Diss. med. vet.

SISSON, S., & J. D. GROSSMAN (1953): The anatomy of the domestic animals. 4th ed. W. B. Saunders Comp., Philadelphia — London

SPURRELL, F. A., L. V. BANDIN & W. F. FELTS (1965): Radiography of the fore limb in the horse. Proc. 11th A. Conv. Am. Ass. Equine Pract., 181

TAVERNOR, W. D., & L. C. VAUGHAN (1962): Radiography of horses and cattle. Br. vet. J. 118, 359

WEBER, W. (1963): Röntgen-anatomische Untersuchungen am Gesichtsschädel des Pferdes. Hannover, Diss. med. vet.

WESTHUES, M. (1942): Die Altersschätzung des Pferdes durch das Röntgenbild der Backenzähne. Tierärztl. Rdsch. 48, 232

ZESKOV, B., J. MAROLT, E. VUKELIC & U. BEGO (1963): Investigations on the radiographical examination of spinous processes in the area of the withers in the horse. Zbl. Vet. Med. A 10, 245

Nachweis entnommener Abbildungen
Sources of illustrations used

Abb./Fig. 1, 3, 7:   WEBER, W. (1963): Röntgen-anatomische Untersuchungen am Gesichtsschädel des Pferdes. Hannover, Diss. med. vet.

Abb./Fig. 33:   HABERMANN, U. (1963): Zur röntgenologischen Darstellung der maxillaren Backenzähne des Pferdes. Hannover, Diss. med. vet.

Abb./Fig. 45, 47:   MEYER, B. (1964): Röntgen-anatomische Untersuchungen am Luftsack des Pferdes. Hannover, Diss. med. vet.

Abb./Fig. 32, 45, 46:   SCHEBITZ, H. (1965): Zur Hemiplegia laryngis (Kehlkopfpfeifen) beim Pferd — Untersuchung und Operationsergebnis. Dtsch. tierärztl. Wschr. 72, 548

Abb./Fig. 64, 65, 69, 70:   SCHEBITZ, H., & H. WILKENS (1965): Zur röntgenologischen Untersuchung des Schultergelenks beim Pferd. Tierärztl. Umschau 20, 486

Abb./Fig. 118, 120:   SCHEBITZ, H., & H. WILKENS (1967): Zum Spat des Pferdes — Untersuchung und Therapie. Berl. Münch. tierärztl. Wschr. 80, 385